Baby and Beyond

Allison Auth

Baby *and* Beyond

Overcoming Those
Post-Childbirth Woes

SOPHIA INSTITUTE PRESS
Manchester, New Hampshire

To my husband and children,
who made me a mother.
Through this journey,
you have shown me the love of God.

Contents

Foreword
by Jenny Uebbing

When I was pregnant with my first child, I expended a *lot* of energy checking off as many of the items on the mommy-to-be to-do list as I could: Bradley classes; breastfeeding prep; reading copious books on topics such as birthing from within, husband-coached childbirth, doula-coached childbirth, unassisted childbirth, water birth, hypnobirthing—all the births!

I spent hours poring over other women's birth stories on the Internet. I took my prenatal vitamins faithfully, hydrated like an elite athlete with my omnipresent Nalgene bottle, drank red-raspberry-leaf tea to tone my uterus, and hired a doula to assist with my planned, unmedicated hospital birth. My patient husband agreed to twelve weeks of childbirth classes and the accompanying instructional videos, which I believe may have scarred him for life.

We had planned for everything.

Except for what actually happened.

My water unexpectedly and definitively broke with a Hollywood-style *pop!* at thirty-seven weeks on the nose, while I sat in the pedicurist's chair at a nail salon.

Baby and Beyond

Huddled in the restroom of the salon, my coworkers nervously pacing in the hallway outside, I panicked. This was not in my birth plan. I was on my lunch break, for goodness' sake! My husband was three suburbs and forty-five minutes away at his office, and I was trapped in the back of Vivi Nails with only a roll of Bounty paper towels and two nervous administrative assistants to help me.

I allowed myself to be coaxed out of the restroom and somehow made it back to the office, where I permitted myself to be driven home, but not before protesting that I was "totally fine!" and could definitely have driven myself.

Once home, I rushed into the bathroom of our tiny apartment and began lighting candles to set the tone for a "positive labor experience." By the time Dave arrived home, he found me sitting in the dark, an overpowering aroma of lavender essential oil in the air as I huddled over a giant exercise ball, moaning in pain, while wax dripped down the side of the tub and onto the floor tiles. He tentatively asked whether it was, perhaps, time to head to the hospital, and I wailed plaintively that we hadn't even had time to use the rolling pin or the tennis balls on my lower back yet.

He must have made a convincing argument, because less than an hour later, I was being wheeled into triage (I had accepted the proffered wheelchair—another failure!) and checked for progress.

"Amniotic fluid confirmed, dilation one … maybe two centimeters. You're on your way to having a baby!"

I was crushed. As the contractions washed over my body, now only three minutes apart, I had been certain I was nearing the transition stage of labor. In reality, my water had broken early, and I was experiencing the pain of a so-called dry labor, a cushion of amniotic fluid no longer easing some of the intensity of the contractions.

But there was more. Nine hours into active labor, I agreed to another cervical exam, thinking surely I was nearing completion. When the nurse straightened up and smiled encouragingly, announcing, "Four centimeters!" I was done. I wept in defeat, my body racked by sobs and contractions. The doula met us at the hospital and patted my back encouragingly, assuring me that I had the strength to continue.

But I didn't.

Defeated, devastated, I yelled our code word for consenting to pain medication. Dave—concerned by my 180-degree turn after a pregnancy spent *adamantly* insisting that I'd do things "my way"—crouched at my bedside and asked, "Are you sure, honey?" Tears of humiliation now mingled with the pain as I nodded furiously, gulping back sobs and begging that he call the anesthesiologist. As he wheeled his cart into the room, I thought I detected a hint of disapproval—or was it disappointment?—in my doula's eyes.

When Joseph Kolbe Uebbing finally made his debut earthside, twenty-one hours after my water had broken, I, too, felt broken. Elated, excited, and in love ... but traumatized by the way his birth had gone. He came into the world sunny-side up—what the medical terminology calls occiput posterior—which is the opposite of the preferred position for birth. He arrived unwillingly after four hours of pushing, the nursing staff glancing anxiously at the clock while my calm, patient doctor assured them that baby was fine and that I could do it.

Baby *was* fine, and I *could* do it—with a little assistance. I ended up with an episiotomy, second-degree tearing, and vacuum assistance, and Joey was dragged into the sunlight with his cord looped tightly around his little neck and torso, making for a tether so short that I could pull him only up to my belly button.

"No wonder he didn't want to come out!" the doctor joked, cutting the cord so that I could lift my sweet, cone-headed baby into my shaking arms. I clutched him to my chest and wept in gladness, in immediate love, and in exhausted pain.

It was nothing like I had imagined. And that discrepancy between expectation and reality would come to haunt me for months.

Our cultural postpartum narrative revolves around an empowered, educated, and highly athletic woman completing pregnancy and childbirth like some kind of endurance event. Much is made of preparing well for the big day, of having the ideal pregnancy, and of achieving the ideal birth experience. My own efforts revolved almost exclusively around preparing for *getting* baby here; very little thought was given to what bringing baby home, and beyond, might look like.

Four days after giving birth, I stood on the sidelines of my husband's rec-league football game, bleeding heavily into a hospital-grade pad, miserably shifting my weight from side to side to alleviate the pain of my stitches. Joey napped in his car seat at my feet while I feigned health and good cheer to his teammates' wives. I had pushed him to go, told him I wanted to be out and about, that having a baby was as natural as breathing, that I was fine! Never mind that I had undergone all manner of unnatural interventions in my birth experience; I could put it all behind me and have the best darn postpartum recovery on record.

I was still trying to "do" motherhood like some sort of adult merit badge, proving to anyone who was watching that I could totally have a baby and jump right back into real life. But I didn't jump back, not really. And a few weeks later, the facade came tumbling down when I was diagnosed with severe postpartum depression. Another notch in my self-assumed belt of failure.

In all the years and babies since, each postpartum period has looked a little different and a little bit the same. The underlying theme of them all? Surrender: to God's plans; to the loss of my plans; to the loss of my expectations and, to a certain extent, my autonomy. There is a beautiful humility to motherhood, if we have eyes to see it. A mother's love is cross-shaped, and our experiences can lead us to the One who has the strength to carry the Cross, if we let Him.

Allison Auth has done a beautiful mercy for mothers everywhere by putting into words how vastly different life after labor can look from what we expect. How I wish I had had her words to accompany and console me during my own "dark nights" of the postpartum soul.

Our culture may be medically and technologically advanced, but we lack the collective wisdom and lived experience necessary to accompany and care well for postpartum mothers. Six weeks of maternity leave and a stack of "body after baby" workout DVDs are not sufficient to address the vastness of what has occurred, to bridge the chasm between *expectant mother* and *mother*.

Physically, mentally, emotionally, spiritually: a baby changes everything. Allison understands this, and she walks the reader bravely through her own experiences of early motherhood, weaving together sound advice, courageous vulnerability, and a rich theological perspective on the sacred, year-long period after birth.

My go-to gift for any new mom, now that I'm a seasoned maternal professional? A month's supply of diapers, a fully loaded coffee gift card, and a copy of this book to reassure her that she is not alone and that her suffering has not been in vain.

May the wisdom to be found here settle deeply into the hearts of all mothers who read it, and may it flow from the maternal heart of Mary, who is Mother to us all.

Baby and Beyond

Why This Book Was Written

I got pregnant when my husband and I were on our honeymoon in Hawaii, and I found out two weeks later after getting nauseated on a roller coaster. I was a youth minister at the time, and on returning from my honeymoon, I took a group of youth to Elitch's amusement park in Denver. I love roller coasters, but after getting off this one, I knew I couldn't do that again. I was on the verge of throwing up and needed to sit down. Could I be pregnant? A few days later, the two lines confirmed that I was.

During that first pregnancy, I read baby books, made my registry list, and set up the nursery. I knew the relative size of my baby each week compared with different fruits and wrote up my natural birth plan. I had read *What to Expect When You're Expecting*, but what I needed to read was *What to Expect When You're Postpartum*.

I was induced at forty-one weeks. After three days in the hospital on an IV drip and a failed induction, I had an emergency C-section. When I packed my bags for the hospital, I figured I didn't need maternity clothes anymore. I had a looser shirt and pants to go home in, but no one told me I'd still look eight months pregnant upon leaving the hospital! I could barely fit those pants over my thighs (let alone button them), and I almost had to wear my bathrobe home! I had been told that nursing would melt the baby fat off, but for me that was not the case. I was wearing maternity clothes for a good three months after my son was born. After that, I had to buy a new wardrobe because none of my prepregnancy clothes fit me.

As with my clothes, I was startled about so many things that occurred during the postpartum time, and for a long while, I felt I must be the only one who experienced them. None of the other mothers I talked to shared about their struggles and insecurities. In the age of comparison, every mother wanted others to see an Instagram-perfect snapshot of her life. They all spoke of how much they loved motherhood, while I felt trapped and overwhelmed by it, not recognizing the person I was before that fated C-section. Of course I loved my baby, but I grieved the loss of my flat tummy, regulated hormones, and freedom to go out at night.

When I found out at nine months postpartum that I was pregnant again, it sent me in a hormonal spiral. Our family was changing faster than I could keep up with, and I didn't know how to adjust to each new challenge. Ever since the birth of my first two children, I have been on a quest to find balance and healing: to recognize motherhood as a holy vocation and to reconcile my physical and emotional struggles as connected in one body-soul union.

I've read many Catholic books on mothering, but none seem to delve deep into the twelve months after having a baby, which I believe is the minimal amount of time to be considered postpartum. The year or so after having a baby is very irregular, particularly difficult, and just plain different from the other years of motherhood. I have often felt guilty about not having the daily schedule and regular prayer routine written about in other Catholic books for moms. I have failed a lot at figuring this mothering thing out, and I want to share with you the lessons I've learned along the way.

One night, while in the shower, I was sharing my thoughts with the Lord, and I heard Him tell me very clearly, "Write a book about postpartum." I reflected on that for a few months, feeling strongly that it was a call from God, but not sure what to do with it. Then a fellow college grad reached out on our household's Facebook page. She had recently had her first child and was diagnosed with postpartum depression. She wrote:

> I don't feel bonded with my baby. At times I feel as if I don't even love her. I know they are all irrational lies but I feel like a horrible mom. [My husband] returns to work Monday and the thought of having to care for her by my-self is so overwhelming and stressful. I don't know what to do. I have wanted to be a mom my entire life and feel like I'm not worthy to be hers cause I'm in such a dark place.

Then, the comments started pouring in:

> Postpartum hormones are no joke! I for sure struggled with two of my kids and it can be isolating and scary.

> You are not alone. I struggled with those exact feelings after each pregnancy, but especially my last one. It was awful and I unfortunately did not get help, which is prob-ably why it lasted well over a year.

> I felt the same way! And honestly I'm glad you posted this because I was afraid to ever tell anyone that I didn't feel bonded/feel love toward my newborn. But taking care of

a newborn (especially your first) IS totally overwhelming and stressful!"

Again and again, moms shared that in their postpartum experiences, they also felt alone, overwhelmed, tired, and guilty. "You are not alone" was the consistent refrain.

And so this book is for you, to help you know that you are not alone. Whether you have full-blown postpartum depression, or simply a roller coaster of other emotions, there is a place for those feelings here. The experiences in this book are mine, but my hope is that in sharing my story, I can offer you some hope and peace for your journey. So grab a cup of coffee or a glass of wine, and read on.

1

Birth Stories

Timothy

At thirty-seven weeks, my OB told me I was three centimeters dilated. I had not felt any contractions, and I was pleasantly surprised that my body seemed built for childbirth. I was told I could have this baby any day! A friend's sister had a later due date than mine, but her baby came three weeks early. A coworker shared that her babies all came three weeks early. It seemed as if I knew a lot of mothers who had their babies weeks before their due dates. I got pregnant so easily that I imagined that birth would be easy, too.

Well, my due date came and went. I walked around the park next to my house, with my shockingly huge belly peeking out beneath my largest maternity shirt. The only shoes that fit were slip-ons, and when walking didn't induce labor, I ran up and down my townhouse stairs in an attempt to jiggle the baby out. Finally, I was induced at forty-one weeks.

After three days in the hospital with a cervix ripener (which did nothing), they broke my water (which also did nothing) and put me on Pitocin. I hadn't even been having noticeable contractions until they started upping the Pitocin to the highest doses. When the contractions finally came, they came in full force, so I asked for an epidural. The needle felt like ice cold steel rubbing against my spine, but immediately relief washed over me — in one leg. That's right, the epidural went in lopsided. While my right side was entirely numb, my left side felt *everything*. A little over twenty-four hours after my water broke, I started to feel feverish, and the doctors decided on an emergency cesarean because I was barely ten centimeters dilated and not fully effaced, and they were worried about the baby.

The nurses gave me medication for my fever, but the medication caused me to shake. My legs and arms were convulsing during the entire surgery, and when my husband put my firstborn son in my arms for the first time, I was shaking so badly that I couldn't hold him. I gave him back to my husband and turned away. In my first official act of motherhood, I turned away from my son, and even though I know the circumstances, it's a moment that has haunted me ever since.

My mom was supposed to return home to watch my sister's kids, but she extended her stay to take care of me after the C-section, since I couldn't drive or even walk upstairs, and my husband had to return to work right away. Two days after we came home from the hospital, I had trouble breathing every time I lay down. My mom took me to the ER, where they performed every test available. I was hooked up and tested for three hours while my mom rocked Timothy in the car seat. If she slowed her rocking, he would start to stir and fuss, and I was in no position to nurse him, so my rock-star mom rocked him for three hours straight (which was probably the cause of her carpal tunnel). In the end, it turned out that I had extra fluid from all my days in the hospital on an IV.

Since I had the shakes right after the C-section and was unable to hold Timothy or nurse him, he was whisked away to have a bottle as his first meal. After that, he was having trouble latching so I had a lactation consultant come to my house and try to help me with different nursing holds. For the first week, I had to pump colostrum and then syringe it into his mouth, and then for the next two weeks I had to use a nipple shield. Even after that, I could only nurse comfortably using a nursing pillow, which made it logistically hard to leave the house.

The one time I did try to leave the house to buy a nursing bra, I drove thirty minutes to a special store and had just stepped into the dressing room when Timothy started screaming to nurse. I sat in the dressing room and nursed him in there for twenty minutes. I unlatched him, but he still wasn't done. I hurriedly bought an overpriced bra and sat in a hot car to finish nursing him for another thirty minutes. It was the most uncomfortable (and most expensive) nursing bra I have ever bought.

Months later, I finally mourned the loss of the birth experience I was hoping for. Although I loved Timothy more than anything, I felt disconnected from him and constantly overwhelmed at each new experience. So getting pregnant again at nine months postpartum was one of the hardest times of my life.

Lily

After my failed induction and long hospital stay with Timothy, I was terrified of giving birth again. It dominated my thoughts and prayers leading up to Lily's birth. Timothy was not quite a year and a half old, and here we were again. I had fears of another C-section; fear of the pain of contractions, failed epidurals, tearing, and stitches. I tried to tell myself over and over again that millions of women have been birthing children for thousands of years, but it wasn't helping. Again, I was three centimeters dilated three weeks before my due date, and again, I had been having no contractions.

My husband, Nathan, was becoming busier with his remodeling business and had landed a big basement finish. He was expecting a large delivery from Home Depot on Friday, November 9, and my due date was November 11. Since Timothy had been so late, I had resigned myself to another past-due baby. Nathan was working hard to get this delivery lined up and told me this baby could come any day that week but Friday.

I was taking a shower late Thursday night when it felt like extra fluid had washed down my legs. It was too hard to tell if that was my water breaking or not, so I got out and got dressed. Over the next half hour, there were more drips in my underwear, and out of caution I called my OB. He was on call overnight at a different hospital from the one I planned on delivering at, but since I wanted to try for a VBAC, I really wanted him to be my doctor. He said to come on in to get examined, so we called the sitter and got ready to head to the hospital. I was going to have this baby on the one day that Nathan had specifically requested I didn't: Friday.

I put a pad in my underwear to catch the slow leak, but that helped only during the car ride. We didn't know that, because of the late hour, we were supposed to enter the hospital through the emergency room, so we walked in through the main entrance, only to have to cross the entire length of the hospital to the emergency entrance. With each step, a little more fluid leaked, and by the time we had reached the emergency room, my pad, underwear, and pants were soaked. They told us to take a seat and wait until they were ready for us. I replied, "Thanks, but I'd rather stand."

A quick test confirmed that it was, in fact, amniotic fluid, and I was admitted even though I wasn't having contractions yet. The fear gripped me as I realized my body was failing at labor once again. The nurses put me on Pitocin and gradually upped the dose all throughout the night, but I still wasn't having any contractions. The next morning came and went, and by the afternoon I was at the highest dose they would allow me on, yet there were no contractions. Crying, I went to the bathroom, sat down, and pushed. It felt like something inside popped, and suddenly the contractions came, long and strong. Totally unprepared, I asked for an epidural. This time it went in smoothly and evenly, and while it brought instant relief, it was not so strong that I couldn't feel the contractions. After the epidural, it took no time to reach ten centimeters, and after a little over an hour of pushing (and a staff shift change), we met our little one.

We hadn't found out the gender ahead of time, so we were eager to find out if our baby was a boy or a girl. As the head came out, I heard the doctor exclaim, "He has so much hair!" I felt very confused because I had been so sure the baby was a girl, but I did not realize her whole body hadn't come out yet. After a few more pushes, there she was, definitely a girl.

Luke

When Lily was eleven months old, I got pregnant again. We didn't have this postpartum NFP thing figured out yet, and it turns out that stress-delayed ovulation is a real thing (so are skewed charts due to nutrient depletion). I took a pregnancy test the day of my brother's wedding, the day my uncle (who is a deacon) reminded me of the blessing for fertility he gave my husband and me on our own wedding day. He said his prayer for fruitfulness was very efficacious, and I would have to agree.

We moved into a fixer-upper when I was eight months pregnant with Luke. It was a raised ranch with two bedrooms on the main level and two bedrooms in the basement. The basement was full of bugs and mice droppings, and my one goal was for Nathan to refinish one of the bedrooms before the baby came. That didn't happen, and so it was going to feel very tight for the five of us to be sharing two small bedrooms.

Again, I had not been having very many contractions, and again I had a fear of labor. I had resigned myself to the fact that I just don't do labor well, and I would be content with whatever interventions were necessary to deliver a healthy baby.

Two days before my due date, I awoke early one morning to a strong contraction. This contraction felt different. It was long, it was strong, and I knew I was in labor. I also knew that contractions were supposed to get closer together, so I climbed back into bed and pulled out my phone. I was really into playing Solitaire at the time, and this morning I was killing it: winning one game after another. I was on a roll, and that's how I knew this was going to be baby day.

Although my contractions were long and strong, they came and went, so I told Nathan to go to work that day. He left for work, and a few hours later, I figured it was time to go to the hospital at least to get checked. My contractions were still sporadic but strong, and since I needed Pitocin the previous times, I suspected that I might need it this time as well. My sister-in-law came over to drive me to the hospital, and Nathan was going to meet me there. It felt so bizarre to wheel my own suitcase into the hospital, walk right up to the desk, and check myself in solo. In the triage room, they hooked me up to the monitor to get a reading on my contractions. A half hour later, there had not been a single contraction. The nurse planned to send me home, but as I stood up, I had a huge contraction while still on the monitor. The nurse finally decided to check me and saw that I was six centimeters dilated. I was staying.

Walking down the halls as I waited for Nathan to arrive helped kick more contractions into gear, but they never got super close together. Again, I had an epidural, but needed no Pitocin this time. That helped me get to ten centimeters quickly and get my contractions a little closer together, but they were never one after another. As with Lily, I had forty-five minutes of pushing that began right at the staff's shift change, so my pushing had to wait until the new nurses were ready. When Luke arrived, I hadn't been at the hospital for even twelve hours. That was a first.

Zoe

Luke was seventeen months old when I got pregnant this time. As I looked at my chart, I couldn't figure out when I had conceived. The chances seemed almost impossible. But if you give God an inch, He'll go a mile, right? I had the most peace with this pregnancy, until about three months before my due date. I no longer feared birth, but I was terrified of the postpartum period. Every time I thought about bringing the baby home from the hospital and the sleepless nights that lay ahead, I cried. I knew I would love this baby and that there would be good moments too, but I allowed the memories of the past and the fear of the future to consume me.

At my thirty-two-week checkup, I took the glucose test and found out I had gestational diabetes. This was odd. With Timothy, my first, I ate donuts for almost my entire pregnancy and passed the glucose test with flying colors. This time around, I ate healthier food than I had with any other pregnancy, and here I was with gestational diabetes. With three kids ages five and under at home and trying to homeschool my kindergartner, it was chaotic. I was having trouble remembering to do anything on a schedule, such as taking my prenatal vitamins. Now I had to record every single thing I ate and take my blood sugar level an hour after eating. How was I going to manage this?

Thanks be to God, He gives graces when we need it. Those eight weeks of diabetes forced me to work on being disciplined about eating, writing down what I ate, and checking my blood sugar. Every day, as I pricked myself, I would think about the blood of Christ. I knew that I was being a wimp about my small cross, but it had more meaning when united to Christ's big one. I began to take my prenatal vitamins more regularly, and I didn't gain as much weight in the last trimester.

Zoe's due date was three days after Christmas. Advent was intense because it was not only preparation for Christmas, but also nesting for myself. We had countdown paper chains hanging from the ceiling, the Advent wreath garnishing our dining table, an Advent calendar from our parish on the windowsill, and a chocolate Advent calendar from my mom (placed out of reach, of course). We did the Jesse Tree and decorated the Christmas tree and wrapped all the presents weeks before Christmas. I was ready. It was also spiritually beautiful to think about walking with Mary and being pregnant during Advent with her. And yet I would cry just thinking about being postpartum.

I was also concerned about being in the hospital on Christmas. I had a very narrow window of time for this baby to be born — while my parents were in town but not while they were skiing and not on Christmas. The first window was a week before

Christmas, and I had been having contractions regularly for days. I knew that they were not labor contractions, but I was hoping they would lead there. (The priests who celebrated Christmas Eve Mass told me afterward that they were thankful I didn't go into labor during Mass, and although I was having contractions the whole time, I was thankful I didn't go into labor then either. A Christmas miracle!)

At thirty-seven weeks, my doctor stripped my membranes, which caused me to go into prodromal labor, meaning I was having regular contractions that are more than Braxton Hicks contractions but not enough to be real labor. And on top of gestational diabetes and three weeks of prodromal labor, I also was so congested that I couldn't breathe through my nose. I tried everything from nasal strips to a humidifier to pseudoephedrine, but nothing helped—nothing save finally giving birth. Also around that time, I contracted a virus that made every muscle in my body weak and painful to move; it was as if my nerves were either cut off from my extremities or going into overdrive. This virus took a full seven days to run its course, and on one of those days, my dear husband, Nathan, had to get me dressed because I could not lift my arms above my waist. I was so ready for birth, but not quite ready for what would come next.

By the time Christmas came, I had already experienced prodromal labor for three weeks, a muscle virus, and lack of sleep from not breathing. My body was extremely sore and tired, and I was exhausted and angry because I still had to go through labor. Two days after Christmas, I woke up experiencing stronger contractions. They were again long and strong, lasting for three minutes, but about ten minutes apart. I had a new OB who didn't know my labor history. Her office was always busy, so I went back and forth for hours about whether I should go to the hospital. My husband worked from home that day, unsure about when to step in. Shortly before lunch, he made me call my OB, and thankfully she said I could come to get checked during the lunch hour. The office was across the street from the hospital, so I came prepared with my hospital bag.

In my head, I crafted a well thought out, passionate speech about why I should be admitted to the hospital and how my contractions never get too close together. I rewrote it a few times in my mind and walked into the doctor's office ready to deliver the speech. Well, I had to stop three times between the parking lot and the waiting room while contractions passed, but then I walked into the doctor's office. The doctor checked me and told me I was four centimeters dilated and fully effaced, so she was happy to admit me. My fears were unfounded, and I had no need for my speech.

We got to the hospital, and I went for the epidural again. My contractions were still logging in at three minutes long and ten to fifteen minutes apart, and I was hoping the epidural would help make them closer together. Nurses busied themselves with getting ready for delivery, and it was approaching dinner and the shift change. Nathan was getting hungry and went to go get something to eat. He told me he would try the hospital cafeteria first, but if nothing looked good he would go to Wendy's. About five minutes after he left, my doctor came in to check me. Lo and behold, I was ten centimeters dilated! I could be ready to push, but if I could wait another ten minutes for the shift change, that would be great. I also needed my husband to be there, so I called his phone, which rang on the table next to me. My doctor graciously went to the cafeteria to check for him, but there was no sign of him. Minutes ticked by, and I was panicking, thinking about my husband missing the birth of our fourth child just for a burger. The minute he walked back in the room, I began to push.

Unfortunately, my contractions still had not come as close together as I would have liked. We were timing my pushes with my contractions, and so there was a considerable length of time between pushes—even as long as five minutes. It was so awkward: my feet in the stirrups, everyone's eyes on me, and nothing was happening. My doctor even checked her phone messages a few times in between pushes. But after forty minutes of intermittent pushing, Zoe was finally here.

I am grateful for the fact that none of our babies had any health issues: no jaundice, no NICU stays, and they even passed their hearing tests with flying colors. I thank God for that gift, because the next stage, going home, was when things got real for me.

2

Postpartum Stories

When I told my parents I was writing a book about my postpartum experiences, my dad remarked, "Ah, so it's a horror story." We all had a good laugh, but the humor is in the irony, because he was partly right. Now, I know not all women will experience difficulties to the degree that I have, but I think each mother will relate to at least one or two. So my hope is that you can gain some insight from my stories in order to overcome your own postpartum woes.

"Postpartum" here refers to the full year after the birth of a child, much longer than the three months usually given for maternity leave or the milestone of the six-week checkup. Marked by sleepless nights, physical recovery, and mental fatigue, postpartum is its own unique aspect of motherhood. So here is a peek into my postpartum life, one child at a time.

Timothy

In those first three months after Timothy's birth, as darkness crept over the horizon, fear crept into my heart. I hated nighttime. Like a wanderer lost in the woods at night, I was desperate to survive the night and make it until morning.

I would rock Timothy in the middle of the night for hours, trying to get him to sleep in his own crib, but he would sleep for only an hour or two at a time. I would swing him back and forth in my arms and angrily whisper, "Shh, shh, shh" while pacing diagonally from one corner of the room to the other. After a few weeks, I knew where all the creaky spots in the floorboards beneath the carpet were and would carefully step to avoid those while pacing the room. Eventually I wore a path in the carpet fibers. I regularly sent this plea up to God: "If this baby doesn't go to sleep soon, *I am going to completely lose it!*" I would repeat that prayer again and again, giving myself just one more time to pace the room before losing it.

After Timothy was born, I didn't leave the house much for the first two months. I vaguely recall my friend Andrea driving me to Target one night a week after I had returned from the hospital and was unable to drive myself yet because of the C-section. I hobbled into Target with my incision still sore, maternity clothes still on, and blinked in the bright lights. I felt as if I were in a weird parallel universe. I had frequented Target often before Timothy was born, but now I felt as if I were walking into the store for the first time. I didn't recognize myself and couldn't reconcile how this was the same me who shopped in this store only two weeks before.

I stood in Target, staring at a wall of Fruit of the Loom underwear. All my underwear had been hitting right at my incision and causing a lot of pain. I was in the market for some granny panties that would go up past my stitches. As I stared and compared and hemmed and hawed, unsure of what size my swollen body currently was, I went for the safest route and got the highest waist I could find in the size larger than what I would normally wear. I felt very confident that my husband wouldn't attempt any funny business while I was wearing those bad boys, and at least they would allow my incision to heal. The big underwear was also great for those thick pads to help with the lochia bleeding that happens for *six weeks after you deliver.* I thought all the blood came out on the delivery table! If somebody had told me about the bleeding beforehand, I sure didn't remember. After not having a period for nine months, it felt unusual to bleed for almost six weeks straight.

I felt so much fear upon doing all the firsts: the baby's first bath, his first haircut, his first steps—those were all my husband's doing. His first bites of food were all a dramatic failure for me, and my diaper bag was overstocked with five outfits and two days' worth of diapers, just in case. I remember getting a pass to the Children's Museum when Timothy was six months old. Two months went by before I gave myself the pep talk of a lifetime just to take my baby somewhere we had never been before.

Around three months postpartum, I had to ease back into my job at the church as a youth minister, which meant working nights and weekends. After I discovered that Timothy preferred sleeping on his belly, sleep returned some of my sanity after holding it hostage for three straight months. My younger sister lived with us that summer and watched Timothy when I went to work, and the arrangement worked pretty well.

When my sister left to return to college, I decided to cut back to working part-time. My training as a catechist wasn't going to pay much—definitely not worth the cost of childcare. I was actually looking forward to spending more time with my son and settling into my role as a mother. I made arrangements with my parish to come in three days a week, from 6:00 a.m. to 9:00 a.m., to do office work, after which I would rush home to take care of Timothy so my husband could go to work. I had a sitter on Fridays, and I worked on Sundays as the director of Confirmation. The schedule reduced the cost of childcare, but it meant that we had less family time, especially if Nathan had to work on a Saturday. When I became pregnant with Lily at nine months postpartum, waking up at 5:30 a.m. to go to work became the hardest thing I ever had to do (okay, besides giving birth), especially since Timothy was still usually waking up to nurse in the middle of the night. I lasted at that job through the school year and quit in June, having four full months at home until my second baby's arrival.

Lily

When our second, Lily, was born, our time in the hospital was magical. Unlike Timothy, I had a vaginal birth, and Lily latched on right away. I no longer had those fears of firsts because I had done this just eighteen months before and knew I could survive. What I didn't know was that there were new experiences to come that would test my limits.

Lily was what you could call colicky. She slept for a solid five hours at a time, but when she was up, she just cried. I even worried that the cops were going to show up at our condo door every time I changed her diaper because of her ear-piercing screams. She hated baths, being buckled into the car seat, and just about anything that wasn't sleeping. She was so stiff that I worried about gas problems and constipation. In those first few months, the only thing that would get her to sleep was manually rocking her in a bouncy seat for a half hour. The thought that got me through that half hour was knowing that she was going to sleep for a long time after.

Meanwhile, we were having nursing problems. Her latch wasn't as magical as I had thought in the hospital, and she was really hurting me. My nipples began to bleed, and layers of my flesh would come off at each feeding. It was so painful that I would end up sobbing on the floor, thinking I couldn't go on living any longer. It didn't just hurt; it was burning through the veins in my chest, and I was pretty sure we both had thrush.

I saw two lactation consultants and tried every position I could. We simply could not get Lily to latch on properly. I told myself we should just give up nursing and use formula, but we were broke, I already had a full supply of milk in my breasts, and formula still wouldn't get rid of our thrush, meaning I would be constantly disinfecting bottles. I was a miserable sort of human being at this point. I told myself that if nursing didn't hurt, I would be fine, but I was only lying to myself. I had postpartum depression, where each day felt like more than a million years long and I wasn't sure I would survive to the next. Someone gave me a six-month outfit when Lily was only a few weeks old. I politely said thanks but in my mind I figured we would never live to see the day when she would fit into it.

Thankfully, I reached out one more time to a lactation consultant, who guessed that the problem might be an upper frenulum lip tie. Apparently, if the skin that attaches the upper lip to the gums is just a little too thick or a little too short, it can cause short-term nursing problems, or even long-term dental problems. She knew of a pediatric dentist at Children's Hospital who had done some research into it and gave me his number. I was desperate to try anything, so a week later, Lily went in for a laser surgery to remove the center fold of skin between her gums and upper lip.

Immediately after the surgery, she began to suck instead of bite at feeding time. A wave of relief washed over me, but it still didn't solve all my problems. It took over a month to heal my nipples, as well as battle our thrush. I tried everything from gentian violet drops (which turn everything purple) to Diflucan and eating an anti-candida diet of strictly meat and vegetables to combat yeast overgrowth, which left me starving. I drank raw apple cider vinegar and applied grapeseed extract on my nipples. I washed all my clothes in hot water and vinegar while doubling down on ibuprofen.

I dreaded the day of Lily's Baptism because I had to be out in public, and I wasn't sure how to nurse her without all my supplies for cleansing and pain management. But I knew that my pain was no excuse for not exercising my duty as a parent to baptize my baby, which washed away her original sin and gave her grace. So, on the Saturday after Christmas, as the deacon poured water over Lily's head, I heard the Lord say to me, "There's a reason she was born. I have a special plan for her." Those words broke through my dull, depressed spirit, and for the first time since her birth, I felt hope. Lily would make it into that six-month outfit after all.

As I began healing over the next several months, I never forgot the struggle of the first three months of Lily's life, which are remembered by Lily's screaming, my crying, and purple, bloody nipples.

Luke

With Luke, our third, I was bound and determined to make up for my postpartum failings of the first two. I wanted to get out of the house every day and take life by the horns. When Luke was two weeks old, my mom came to visit, and we went to the railroad museum in the next town over. All the rail cars were sitting outside in a yard, it was over ninety degrees, and I was sweating with Luke on my chest in the carrier. I had to sit down several times to rest because I was in pain from the stitches where I tore during the birth.

When Luke was six weeks old, some family came for his Baptism, and I wanted to show them a good time. I planned splash pads, museums, and even a drive up to the peak of Mount Evans, the highest paved road in America. It didn't occur to me until we got there that, at over fourteen thousand feet, this elevation wasn't great for Luke's newborn lungs. I spent most of that afternoon nursing him in the car while everyone else explored. He was so sleepy, and I was afraid he wasn't getting enough oxygen, so I was relieved finally to make it down the mountain.

On top of that, we invited a fourteen-year-old French relative of mine to stay with us for three weeks that summer. At the time, it seemed like a great idea, since she could play with the two- and three-year-old while I nursed the baby. She was wonderful, and play with them she did, but I also felt obligated to show her Denver, since she had traveled a third of the way around the world to come here. So we explored the foothills, drove up mountains, went to pools, visited museums, and so forth.

Meanwhile, my husband was working hard, nights and weekends, to set up his shop and make our house more inhabitable. From water leaks and mold, to musty carpets and bad wiring, there was always something to work on. Not only were we physically exhausted from having three kids in four years, moving to a fixer-upper, growing Nathan's business, and hosting a foreign relative, but we were also emotionally taxed from all that that entailed.

A week or so after Segolene had returned to France, my muscles ached, and I could barely move. I remember being at a baby shower and trying not to sit down, because if I did, I feared my body would shut down for good. I hadn't used the last three months after having a baby to rest, and now I was feeling it. My body was yelling at me to slow down.

Another postpartum difficulty with Luke was his reflux. It didn't happen after every feeding, but often during morning feedings. There was an abundance of spit-up all day long, but a few feedings a day were followed by projectile vomiting. Luke even vomited once in the pediatrician's office, but the doctor didn't have any recommendations for me that I hadn't tried. Looking back, perhaps I could have cut out dairy or tried a formula, but since it was usually the morning feedings, I assumed it had to do with overeating after sleeping for ten hours straight. Yes, this kid started sleeping through the night at around eight weeks old. But when he was awake, he was a spit-up master. When I heard the familiar gagging noise, I ran to the hardwood floor so that it would be easier to clean up than on the carpet. There was no trying to contain it with a blanket because there was no telling how far it would go.

Because of this, I tried diligently to time our outings with nursing so that we wouldn't have to do morning feedings on the go; I would rather clean up the projectile mess in our own house. But one Sunday morning, when Luke seemed to be going through a feeding spurt, he again became hungry during the Liturgy of the Eucharist, even though I had nursed him right before Mass. I went to the cry room to nurse him quickly so I could go up to Communion with the rest of my family. As we walked up the aisle, I held Luke very carefully so as not to jostle him. Unfortunately, it didn't matter. About three people away from receiving the precious Body of Christ, my precious little one projectile-vomited all over me and the lady in front of me, just two steps away from the priest. Everyone in the front row got a good view of the show, which, luckily, included the parish janitor. The front of my shirt was soaked with milk, as well as the back of the blouse of the middle-aged lady in front of me.

I ran to hide in the bathroom while my husband apologized profusely to the victim of the crime. She just happened to be in the wrong place at the wrong time: in line for Communion. Fortunately, she was understanding and assured me she remembered those days when her kids were babies. Thank God for small miracles!

When Luke was three months old, I saw an ad in our parish's bulletin for a hospitality coordinator. The ad caught my eye, since I used to work for the church and that line of work was familiar to me. The job was only on Sundays, so it wouldn't interfere with my husband's job. We needed more money, so I applied. During the job interview, I was asked if I was the one whose baby threw up in the line for Communion, and I sheepishly owned up to it. The parish gave me the job anyway!

The part-time job went well for a few months, until our family life fell apart. Between Nathan's job, my part-time job, working on our house, and having three kids five and under, we were spent. A few months later, I began to experience what I call an emotional breakdown, and by June I quit my job. The telltale sign that I wasn't doing too well: on my last day of work at the church, after being there for several hours, I looked down to discover I had two entirely different sandals on.

When Luke was eleven months old, my fertility began to return, and my anxiety ramped up. I was now working a new part-time job from home, doing online marriage prep, and the learning curve was steep. I was constantly either yelling at the kids or sticking them in front of the TV. I felt so paralyzed that I could barely make decisions, and I began to have panic attacks. One time, I even had to pull over while I was driving because the panic was so palpable: my heart was racing, my breath escaping in short bursts, and my vision became blurred.

This emotional breakdown was due to a combination of factors: circumstances, stress, vitamin deficiency, and fluctuating hormone levels. I could tell that my body was trying to restart cycles of fertility, and after a few months, when my hormone levels eventually stabilized and my period returned, I noticed that I began to feel a little more even-keeled.

Zoe

The fourth time's a charm, in some respects. I had spoken with my doctor, who is also a mother, about my fears of postpartum. I cried every time I talked about what life might be like after Zoe's birth. When I went to the doctor for Zoe's two-week checkup, I got a shot of progesterone, which can help with postpartum depression. I didn't feel at that moment that I needed it, but I wasn't going to miss the opportunity, as I had all the other times. Whether it helped or not, I do not know. While some mothers experience postpartum depression right off the bat, mine is usually a gradual experience that develops over time.

This time around, my husband and I were in a good rhythm. He knew how to pitch in and help out, and I knew to verbalize my needs and warn him when I was on the verge of a meltdown. I knew that nursing would hurt for the first few weeks, regardless of what I did, and kept up on my ibuprofen. I was okay with the kids watching TV while I was nursing. I gave birth two days after Christmas, so we hunkered down for the winter and enjoyed the kids' new Christmas toys. Friends brought meals, and I invited them to stay for some company. I had started a new vitamin regimen while pregnant with Zoe, and this seemed to help with my mood and recovery (more on that in chapter 4). I was homeschooling my oldest, so while Zoe was napping in the morning, we would read by the fire, play math games, or do crafts.

A few other factors that made the postpartum time after Zoe's birth different was that I didn't have thrush, she was a good sleeper (sleeping through the night at eight weeks old), and she was not a puker, like her brother. These circumstances definitely made postpartum life a lot more bearable!

And yet I was back at the doctor's around eleven months postpartum because I was having a breakdown similar to the one I had when Luke turned eleven months old. Zoe wasn't sleeping through the night anymore, thanks to teething. My voice was hoarse from yelling at the kids. I was stressed about finances. My husband was working very hard, but I felt as if I needed so much from him. I was angry, scared, and anxious. I couldn't lose the baby weight. I would feel sad in the middle of the day for no apparent reason; I felt like a shell of the person I had been before I had kids, and I wondered, "How did I end up here?"

3

Postpartum Depression and Depletion

At my children's two-week checkups, I was usually asked, "Do you want to hurt yourself or your baby? No? Okay, good. Do you cry all the time? No? Okay, good." And that was that.

I had heard about postpartum depression and the "baby blues," but what no one ever told me is that there is a real range of emotions that comes after a baby is born. Some experiences are circumstantial: *if only Lily wasn't biting me while nursing; if only I was getting more than two hours of sleep at a time.* Others are purely hormonal: *something just feels off.*

What I discovered was that I don't really experience depression and baby blues as simply defined. But I do experience a fluctuation of unexplained sadness, crippling anxiety, and uncontrollable rage. And after having four children, I know that this experience is definitely related to postpartum.

Many other mothers I know have some difficulty in coping during this time of transition, and some are reluctant to call it depression but don't know what else to call it.

The Postnatal Depletion Cure

One fall, my friend and I signed up for a women's retreat. When we arrived on Saturday morning, we discovered that it was a silent retreat, but I welcomed the silence, and the fact that I hardly knew anyone else made it easier. Lunch was awkward, though, sitting in a crowded cafeteria while eating in silence. I recognized the woman next to me as a physical therapist whom a friend had highly praised for helping with physical recovery after birth. I made the decision to break the silence rule in order to introduce myself. I am so glad I did, because we had such an inspiring conversation about postpartum recovery. I shared with her that I was having a hard time finding answers to connect all my mental and physical difficulties of recovery. She told me she was reading a book called *The Postnatal Depletion Cure* that had been released earlier that year and highly recommended it.

I checked the book out of the library and found the first six chapters immensely helpful. The book's author, Dr. Oscar Serrallach, found that in his professional experience, most modern postpartum care is centered on the baby with only a nod to the mother. There is relatively little literature on topics such as the effects of vitamin deficiencies and hormone imbalances in a postpartum woman. In his personal experience, Dr. Serrallach noticed that his partner, with whom he had three kids, suffered brain fog, loss of confidence, a feeling of isolation, extreme fatigue, and anxiety, and was not fully able to take care of herself and the kids. She had a deep fear that she would never recover or feel the same again. And I could relate.

From his experience as a doctor and his years of research and treatment of postpartum women, he noticed that vitamin deficiency, sleep deprivation, lack of community and time for self-care, the need for physical recovery, and the struggle of adjusting with a partner or spouse all contributed to what he called a mother's "postnatal depletion." I loved that the author saw how all the pieces of the puzzle contribute to this syndrome and then took steps to address each facet of recovery. From his book I gained some valuable information, such as that in order to improve my hormone levels, I first had to rebuild my supply of micronutrients (vitamins and minerals) that years of pregnancy and breastfeeding had left me depleted in.

In addition, I learned that the average prenatal vitamin is designed to give the mother what she needs to keep the baby healthy, but often not enough for the mother herself. So I started to look for high-potency, food-based vitamins, without any fillers, that would help me absorb the most nutrients. The main micronutrients that women are commonly deficient in are iron, zinc, vitamin D, all the B vitamins, and magnesium, which are pretty important ones for basically every cellular function. And it turns out feet are really good at absorbing magnesium, so I bought a bag of Epsom salt (magnesium sulfate) and treated myself to a weekly twenty-minute foot soak!

Postpartum Depression

In his book, Dr. Serrallach also mentioned the difference between postpartum depression and postpartum depletion. Postpartum depression (PPD) is a mood disorder that sets in within the first few months after giving birth. The extreme sadness, anger, and anxiety of depression make it difficult for a mother to care for herself or her baby. Depletion, on the other hand, is a lesser condition, often called the "baby blues," in which hormone deficiency, anxiety, or brain fog results when a mother does not restore her supply of vitamins and minerals that she has given to her baby through pregnancy or nursing.

When Luke was born, I would characterize my experience as depletion, since my emotions were like a roller coaster, with highs and lows. The more I took my supplements and the more sleep I got, the better I felt. With Lily, though, there was no joy. Every day seemed like a thousand years, and I wasn't sure there would be a tomorrow. I didn't gaze on my baby with smiles and flutters; I simply dutifully took care of her. I couldn't see how bad it was, and no amount of sleep would help. I shut out my husband and son and turned inward to conserve energy, but that just led to isolation and more hopelessness. That was a case of postpartum depression, which current statistics suggest about 15 percent of women experience.

Some of the characteristics of depression include struggling to get out of bed, difficulty concentrating, sadness for no apparent reason, low self-esteem, changes in eating and sleeping, and wanting to harm yourself or others.

When I went to my doctor at eleven months postpartum with Luke, I was given a test called the Edinburgh Postnatal Depression Scale. It asked whether I was able to laugh or find enjoyment in things, whether I had difficulty sleeping, whether I had difficulty coping, whether I felt sad or miserable, and other such questions. But it also asked whether I blamed myself unnecessarily when things went wrong, or felt scared or anxious for no good reason, or felt overwhelmed. Based on those criteria, I did fit the bill for a depression diagnosis.

What I have been learning since then is that many forms of postpartum depression and anxiety have their roots in nutritional and hormonal depletion, and if these nutrients are not replenished, the effects could last for years after the birth of your baby.

Consider that all the vitamins and minerals your developing baby received to grow in utero were donated from your body. Combined with the life changes and sleep deprivation of motherhood, of course it takes its toll on your body and your brain!

Luckily, many doctors are now recognizing that progesterone easily bottoms out after labor, and sometimes all a mother might need is a few doses of progesterone to be back on her feet again. Unfortunately, there are still countless doctors who don't even offer progesterone shots as an option, and I've heard stories of women who have had to self-advocate for this treatment in their precarious postpartum condition. Yet studies show the dramatic decrease of postpartum symptoms after progesterone therapy. It seems that one of the reasons progesterone bottoms out is the lack of vitamins and minerals needed to restore hormone balance. In addition, "stress itself uses up more of all the nutrients needed to keep the body working smoothly, particularly the B vitamins, vitamin C, essential fatty acids, and key minerals like zinc and magnesium."[1]

Postpartum depression can also be compounded by a variety of factors. With Lily, it was not only depletion contributing to my depression, but also painful nursing, a colicky baby, having a toddler in the house, and the stress and financial strain of my husband's starting his own business. I couldn't see the light at the end of the tunnel, and I couldn't get a grip on the swirl of emotions raging inside me—sadness, anger, hopelessness, and anxiety on repeat.

One example that stands out was during Advent, when Lily was a month old and Timothy was nineteen months old. I had

---

[1] Dean Raffelock and Robert Rountree, *A Natural Guide to Pregnancy and Postpartum Health*, with Virginia Hopkins and Melissa Block (New York: Penguin Putnam, 2002), 6.

gone upstairs to put Lily down in her swing and was up there for maybe ten minutes. We had been lighting our Advent wreath every night with matches, and somehow Timothy got hold of the giant box of matches and had lit one of them. I heard crying and came downstairs to a smoldering box of matches and a small hole burned in the carpet on the bottom step, where Timothy had burned his fingers and dropped the matches. I have no idea why the fire wasn't bigger, and I credit our guardian angels for that. After first having concern for Timothy, I felt rage toward Nathan. I called him up and yelled into the phone, "*You are the worst father ever!* You are *never* supposed to teach your children how to play with matches!" I wish I could take those words back, and I'm glad that Nathan can laugh about it now. But I was in such a dark place that I alternated between sadness and rage almost constantly.

At about four or five months postpartum with Lily, life began to look more hopeful. As the weather started warming up, it seemed as if I did too. I remember taking Lily outside on our back patio one evening and sitting next to her in the bouncer, watching Timothy and Nathan shoot hoops in the Little Tykes basketball net. It was the first time we had all hung out outside as a family, and I was smiling and laughing and thinking to myself, "Finally, this is what motherhood should feel like."

Depletion

In those suffering depletion of vitamin and mineral stores, depressive or anxious feelings can occur. Different from the inability to get out of bed or the desire to hurt oneself or others, depletion can manifest itself as bouts of sadness, anxiety, or anger. Mothers have also used the terms "weepy," "foggy," or "fearful" to describe the challenges of their emotional state after their babies were born. Often the feelings come and go, and they are not usually crippling. The symptoms may worsen over time, though, if nutrient stores are not replenished through a good diet and vitamin supplements.

I struggled with various types of anxiety and fear of social situations, but I knew I really had a problem when going to my moms' group—a gathering I had loved and looked forward to—began to cause anxiety. I began to avoid going out with other moms, responding to texts, or making phone calls to set up doctor appointments because it felt too overwhelming. What once was manageable now became unbearable partly because I was furthering my depletion.

So, while I struggled with anxiety as well as feelings of sadness after Luke and Zoe were born, I would categorize them as depletion. I was struggling, but I was aware that I was struggling, and in between, there were joyful moments, such as baby snuggles and smiles. I still had some hope that I'd get a handle on my emotions eventually. It was only after Luke and Zoe approached their first birthdays that my condition worsened to the point where I needed help.

Nutrients for Recovery

When I went to my first appointment at the women's natural care clinic at eleven months postpartum with Luke, I burst into tears as the nurse practitioner listened attentively to my struggles with anxiety and depression. A blood draw revealed that I was severely low in vitamin D, and some of my other vitamin levels were pretty low as well. That was my first lesson in not buying cheap, store-brand vitamins! And for some reason, at least here in

Denver, most women are deficient in vitamin D, so that became a regular supplement in my pillbox.

At a different appointment, a test done by my chiropractor showed that my zinc levels were low as well. After having three babies in a row and nursing for five years without good vitamin supplements, I was depleted. I was giving all the good stuff to my children without restoring my own levels. Then a friend of mine who was a nurse and suffered severe postpartum depression (PPD) with her first four children told me that supplementing with fish oil, vitamin D, and vitamin B was a huge factor in her not having PPD with her fifth and sixth children. It turns out that omega-3s are not only good for your heart and brain but are a mood booster as well. A study that examined fish consumption and the incidence of postpartum depression in several different countries found that the more fish women ate, the less likely they were to develop PPD.

When I was pregnant with Zoe, I began taking probiotics in addition to my prenatals, vitamin D, and fish oil. I cried at the cost of forking over precious budget money for vitamins, but I needed to feel better. I decided to forgo the zinc and vitamin B at this time, but after Zoe was born, I saw that they also were necessary supplements for my condition. From there, I began a journey to learn why these vitamins were so important to my health.

The Answer to Prayers

"The well-nourished person can perform a tremendous amount of work, day in and day out, without reaching 'wit's end.' Cutting down on caffeine is the first step because it contributes to that anxious feeling. The mineral magnesium is probably the most noticeable nerve-calming nutrient, followed by the B vitamins, especially B6, vitamin C, zinc, and flax oil."[2]

I was complaining to a friend that I felt off. Even when the baby was sleeping through the night, I still woke up tired. My exhaustion was leading to more anxiety and depression. I felt this disconnect between my body and my soul, and I told my friend that if I just knew what to do, I'd do it!

After a particularly difficult week, I was at Sunday Mass, begging God for joy. It was Gaudete Sunday, during Advent, the pink-candle Sunday of joy, and I felt I had none. The words of the Eucharistic prayer seemed especially poignant that day: "As we wait in joyful hope for the coming of our Savior, Jesus Christ."

I was disappointed when I didn't magically feel more joyful after Mass, but I know that God usually doesn't work that way. Instead, I found myself opening *Fertility, Cycles, and Nutrition* by Marilyn Shannon, a book I had on my shelf since the beginning of my marriage but hadn't read much of. A Catholic who began researching the connection between nutrition, health, and fertility decades ago, Marilyn Shannon has continued to update her book in several editions over the years as more research has become available. I had always considered it a Natural Family Planning book, since it is published by the Couple to Couple League, an NFP organization, but I never considered the book for postpartum.

I found in there a wealth of information that confirmed other postpartum-book findings, plus some simple things to try to improve my physical health. For example, I had wondered if my vivid dreams were causing me to be tired when I woke up, and

---

[2] Marilyn M. Shannon, *Fertility, Cycles, and Nutrition*, 4th ed. (Cincinnati: Couple to Couple League International, 2009), 57.

I found that taking my vitamins before bed was likely part of the cause. I was taking my vitamins at night because I had a full belly and it was the only time I seemed to be able to remember to take them, but once I started taking my vitamins in the morning, the vivid dreams stopped, and I felt (slightly) more rested come morning. I was able to cut back to one cup of coffee in the morning since caffeine can contribute to anxiety (although when the babies were little and I wasn't getting a lot of sleep, I did depend on two or three cups).

Another symptom I noticed was that I felt lightheaded in the morning after eating food with added sugar (even yogurt or toast). Marilyn Shannon talked about blood glucose levels and how high levels cause the adrenal glands to emit more stress hormones. She said that if you wake up tired and aren't hungry first thing in the morning, you could have a blood glucose problem. An easy fix for this is to cut out sugar and empty carbs, such as waffles and dinner rolls, and to eat more whole grains, fruits, and vegetables. Although the idea is simple, the execution was much more difficult. But I found echoing in my head the words I had told my friend: "If I just knew what to do, I'd do it!"

The common thread underlying my symptoms was that my vitamin and mineral deficiency led to abnormal hormone levels, which led to anxiety, fatigue, and constant stress. My consistent mental or physical stress (including nutrition depletion, lack of sleep, mental anxiety, allergies, and so forth) was taking an incredible amount of energy from my body, and as a result, my adrenal glands were underproducing. Here are some of the other sentences from the book that stood out to me:[3]

---

[3] Ibid., 185–186.

Mood swings, anxiety, and low energy can also be improved by nutrition bolstering the function of the adrenal cortex.

Nourishing the adrenal glands pays off well with calmer nerves, improved sexual desire, and normal levels of estrogen in the body.

The adrenal glands need a variety of nutrients: vitamin A, the B vitamins, especially pantothenic acid, plenty of vitamin C, vitamins D and E, and the minerals magnesium, zinc, and manganese. They must have an adequate supply of the essential fatty acids to produce their hormones.

All these vitamins not only support the adrenal glands, but all your hormone levels, including thyroid, DHEA, estrogen, and progesterone.

Among the many tasks they perform, adrenal cortical hormones also keep blood glucose levels up between meals. Because low blood glucose can make it difficult to concentrate, attention to the nutritional needs of the adrenals will help prevent the common complaint of "brain fog."

The simplest answer became clear. Working to restore my body would help my anxiety as well. I felt that God was answering my prayer by giving me the first step to joy. If I could feel more well-rested and less foggy-brained, I could turn my attention to my mental and spiritual health. Thus, I began to read another book, *A Natural Guide to Pregnancy and Postpartum Health,* which Marilyn Shannon recommended in her book.

As I read more, a picture began to emerge of the hormones that affect postpartum women. Thyroid hormone, cortisol, prolactin, progesterone, and estrogen can all influence a woman's emotional state. Feeling tired, anxious, depressed, and wearing mismatched sandals could be the results of a number of imbalances.

This is where I found myself. I knew that being on the SSRI Zoloft had really helped me, but the feeling had started to plateau, and I didn't want to be dependent on it long term if there are other factors at play, such as nutrient depletion. The medicine kept my anxiety in check, but I still felt sad and tired.

I knew that vitamins wouldn't solve all my problems, but since we are body-soul unions, it was worth looking into. So I dug further into details about the roles of vitamins and hormones.

B Vitamins

B vitamins are involved in making just about every hormone and neurotransmitter, so they are important for everything from progesterone levels to serotonin. A B-complex supplement can also help if you suffer from depression, fatigue, or headaches.

Vitamin D

Most people know that vitamin D helps with the absorption of calcium and is therefore good for your bones. But vitamin D also helps with the absorption of iron, magnesium, phosphate, and zinc and aids cells in getting their jobs done. Muscle weakness, lower backache, and frequent or recurrent infections could all be symptoms of low vitamin D.

Magnesium and Zinc

Seventy-five to ninety-five percent of people who are tested are shown to be magnesium deficient. Like zinc, magnesium plays a role in more than three hundred reactions at the cellular level. Bone health, heart health, muscular relaxation, and digestion are processes that require magnesium and zinc to function. Depression, fatigue, menstrual cramps, high blood pressure, and migraines can all be symptoms of low zinc or magnesium.

Trace Minerals

Trace minerals such as manganese, selenium, molybdenum, iodine, and copper are required for healthy hormone function (such as thyroid), metabolism, and blood-sugar control. Selenium is also needed for serotonin production. These trace minerals are important for brain function, mood control, and how histamines are metabolized, "which, in turn, affects allergies, skin rashes, and eczema."[4] A good multivitamin should have adequate levels of these, so check your labels.

DHEA

DHEA is a hormone produced by your adrenal glands. It's the precursor for estrogen and testosterone. "DHEA plays roles in immune function, adaptability to stress, heart function, libido, and mood. Your body cannot make adequate amounts of DHEA or other adrenal hormones without enough vitamin B3, vitamin B6, vitamin C, pantothenic acid, manganese, zinc, and essential fatty acids."[5]

Thyroid

If you are depressed and tired, are gaining weight, are losing hair, or have dry skin, low thyroid function might be the reason. The thyroid helps regulate metabolism, muscle control, mood, heart, and digestive function. The prevalence of hypothyroidism in

---

[4] Oscar Serrallach, *The Postnatal Depletion Cure* (New York: Grand Central Life and Style, 2018), 72.
[5] Raffelock and Rountree, *Natural Guide to Pregnancy*, 187.

postpartum women has skyrocketed in the last twenty years or so, but there's not a clear reason why. It's possible that one factor is that we have less iodine in our diets, as the thyroid needs iodine, in addition to other vitamins, in order to function.

"Thyroid hormones regulate how much oxygen the cells receive, so they increase mental alertness and have potent effects on mood and energy levels."[6]

Progesterone

Progesterone is a calming, protecting, balancing hormone. It plays many roles in the body, such as relieving anxiety, normalizing blood sugar and zinc and copper levels, helping thyroid function, helping the body use fat for energy, and working with estrogen for reproductive function.

> With many of the women we treat for postpartum ailments, hormone testing shows that estrogen production is not significantly low, but progesterone is bottomed out. These two hormones are meant to strike a balance; their effects are complementary. This imbalance can cause a wide range of symptoms, including anxiety, depression, fatigue, foggy thinking, insomnia, irritability, and weight gain. An estrogen/progesterone imbalance can also disrupt the function of thyroid hormones and of cortisol, which is produced by the adrenal glands. A course of supplemental natural progesterone can correct this imbalance.[7]

By the end of my research, I was feeling better, but I knew there was still a missing piece. I had been taking all the vitamins,

[6]   Ibid., 191.
[7]   Ibid., 187.

trying to exercise, and getting a good night's sleep, yet I was still tired all the time. And when I'm tired, I'm sad. Thus, the exhaustion and lightheadedness led me to look closer at my thyroid levels. Although I was told they were in the normal range, my T3 and T4 levels were really more low than normal. I guessed that I was probably lightheaded because my body wasn't metabolizing my food properly, leading to blood glucose and cholesterol problems, along with the inability to lose weight. After convincing my doctor with paragraphs of research on the benefits of thyroid medicine at my levels, she wrote me a prescription for NP Thyroid tablets. It felt like the missing piece and my answer to prayers; it has made a big difference in my energy levels and metabolism, in turn boosting my mood and mental capacity.

Essential Fatty Acids

I was told to take omega-3s while I was pregnant because they were good for my baby's developing brain, and I did take them when my friend told me they helped her avoid having postpartum depression, but I was surprised when I learned more about how essential fats really are. In fact, the human brain is more than 60 percent fat! Fats are necessary building blocks for hormones and energy production.

"Messengers called prostaglandins that regulate important processes throughout your body — including immune-system and reproductive function, the inflammatory response, the constriction and expansion of blood vessels, and blood clotting — are made exclusively from fats."[8]

When you are pregnant, you need not only enough fats to build your baby's brain and body but enough to keep *your* brain

[8]   Ibid., 51.

and body working as well. "The placenta draws DHA from the mother's body like a vacuum cleaner, and the milk ducts continue to drain her stores for as long as her baby nurses," say the authors of A Natural Guide to Pregnancy; and "if you do not keep replenishing your supply, your emotional and physical well-being will most likely be compromised in the postpartum period and beyond."[9]

In fact, some research shows that women who are deficient in EPA and DHA are six times more likely to develop serious mental disorders, such as depression and obsessive-compulsive disorder, and that risk remains higher for two years after giving birth.[10] When I read that, I was floored, because it was always around eleven months after birth and eleven months of nursing that I landed in the doctor's office for depression and anxiety.

There are two big categories of essential fatty acids—omega-6 and omega-3. They are both important as long as they are in balance with one another. A typical American diet is loaded with omega-6s (the "bad," inflammatory ones), while omega-3s (ALA, EPA, and DHA) are found in fewer foods. Fish is a good source of omega-3s, but I hate fish and didn't want to eat it three times a week, so I went the supplement route, while also eating more flaxseed, avocados, and whole-milk dairy.

"Research studies have shown that problems as varied as asthma, autoimmune diseases, depression, skin problems, and emotional ups and downs may improve when a healthy fatty acid balance is restored."[11]

In the end, I wish I could say that my supplements and thyroid medication have magically changed me and that now I'm

[9] Ibid., 97.
[10] Ibid.
[11] Ibid., 52.

healthy and happy all the time. They have greatly reduced my PMS, regulated my cycles, and helped me not to have any more emotional breakdowns. But they did not automatically make me joyful each morning when I woke up. I have to choose joy, and I still have to make the effort to choose to eat healthy foods in addition to my supplements. Supplements can make up for where our diet is lacking, and overcome depletion from pregnancy and nursing, but they are not a replacement for healthy eating.

4

Physical Recovery

When I was working as a course instructor for CatholicMarriage-Prep.com, couples would fill out worksheets, and I would review them and return to them an answer key. One of the most profound ideas that those answer keys taught me was the importance of the body. What we do with our bodies and how we take care of them matters greatly.

After my youngest child, Zoe, was born, my body was a mess. I couldn't stand up straight, all my joints were achy, and I suffered from fatigue and anxiety. I realized that if I wanted my body to reflect God's presence in me, I needed to take care of that body and figure out what it would take to restore it. What I've come back to again and again is that you are what you eat.

Diet

"The ideal diet for a woman recovering from depletion includes moderate to high levels of fat, moderate levels of protein, and small amounts of carbohydrates in her meals every day."[12]

[12] Serrallach, *Postnatal Depletion Cure*, 81.

I'm a sucker for baked goods. During my first pregnancy, with Timothy, I craved donuts all the time. It was my Monday-morning tradition to pick up a donut on my way home from my prenatal appointment. After Timothy was born, I took up baking as a hobby to do while he was sleeping. Cakes, cookies, scones—you name it, I baked it. When I had gestational diabetes with Zoe and couldn't eat sugar, I looked forward to the day, after delivery, when I could finally eat a cinnamon roll.

Over the course of my postpartum journey, I have found it valuable to pay attention to my diet. I love sugar, but I know that eating it exacerbates my physical and emotional problems. I learned a lot after Lily was born about necessary nutrients and vitamins in whole, unprocessed foods. Unfortunately, refined sugar, flour, processed foods, and hydrogenated oils all further hormone imbalance, inflammation, and depletion. Therefore, the less sugar I eat, the less moody I am and the better digestion I have. So now my goal is to eat as fresh as possible and avoid as much processed food as possible. And I've learned to read the labels on the premade food I do buy!

Although I struggle to cut out sugar, I realize that I need more healthy fats for the reasons mentioned in the last chapter. I think that's why Marilyn Shannon recommends flax oil or fish oil for just about every ailment covered in her book. A lowfat diet will also be low in the essential fatty acids and amino acids required for brain and nervous system function, and more likely to be high in sugar. Eating simple carbohydrates (where you burn sugar) keeps your stress systems hyperactive and can lead to inflammation.

"Low or no-grain diet will lead to less inflammation, is more nutrient dense, and leads to more stable blood sugars."[13] So, if

[13] Ibid., 91.

you need a place to start, as I did, there it is: more healthy fats, less sugar and carbs, lots of vegetables and lean meat.

Still, I am realistic and don't agonize over every food choice. I have found that when I slack on my diet and eat more sugar and carbs over a period of time, I feel the negative effects of it and need to get back on track. But that doesn't mean I can't enjoy a dessert here or there: it's all about balance. As a priest once said, "We are Catholic, so food and drink are part of the equation. We are meant to enjoy food, not obsess over it. But know what foods take care of your body."

My relationship with food is changing over time because, although I'm used to indulging my cravings, I'm trying to find that balance between enjoying food and being disciplined. I have not always had good discipline in my eating habits, but my stint with gestational diabetes gave me the chance to work on that. And I do believe that having a level of discipline when it comes to food helps you to have discipline in other areas of life. It's part of the reason we fast during Lent. It's a discipline I struggle with, but I have hope that I can continue to work on it over time — at the very least, for forty days before Easter each year.

Gas

I walked into my six-weeks-postpartum doctor's visit with a long list of items to discuss. This was my fourth time postpartum in six years, so, on the one hand, I had been through this before and knew what felt different from other recoveries, and on the other hand, my body seemed to hurt more and recover more slowly with each delivery.

The various obstacles to my postpartum recovery were not glamorous, and, in fact, were quite embarrassing for me to bring up, even to my doctor. I took a deep breath and began explaining to the RN (whom I had never previously seen for any prenatal appointments):

"My constipation is still really bad, even though I'm drinking what feels like gallons of water every day. And I have really bad gas. I mean, really bad. Also, the site where I tore and have stitches is still really sore and tender."

Her answer? "Your body goes through a lot of trauma during pregnancy and delivery. All your organs are getting squished and shifted around. It takes nine months to grow a baby and nine months to recover. Give your body some time and drink even more water."

In some ways, that was helpful, but in most ways, it wasn't. I thought I had been drinking gallons of water, but I was still constipated. I was taking fiber gummies and probiotics, but the gas remained.

Often, since I was usually holding Zoe, I could try to blame the smell on her. More often, I just tried not to go anywhere. One winter night, I hurriedly ate dinner and took my husband's truck to pick up my friend on our way to our women's prayer group. On my way over, the gas began. We were fairly new friends, and I was so nervous to be stuck in the truck with her for twenty minutes, because there was no way to avoid the smell. I didn't even want to be in the truck with myself, the smell was so bad! I rolled down the windows and reached around my husband's console until I found some of his masculine-smelling lotion. I rubbed it all over my arms and hands, hoping to help mask the smell. As my friend got into the truck, I decided to come clean and, ahem, clear the air. I told her that an unfortunate consequence of postpartum had been really bad gas and that I was so sorry, but I would leave the windows cracked even though it was ten degrees outside. I held my breath and waited for her to ask me to turn around so she could drive herself.

All she said was, "Oh, that's okay. I'm doing a Whole 30 right now, and eating a lot of vegetables and fruits has made me really gassy, too. So you're in good company."

After that, there wasn't anything we couldn't talk about. At around three months postpartum, the gas left for good.

Pain

By six months postpartum, I had made another appointment with my doctor's office. I still had vaginal pain. As the nurse practitioner examined me, she described what she said looked like rings of blisters. I concurred that that's what it felt like. It was still extremely sensitive in the area where I had stitches from tearing as well. She had me make another appointment with my delivery doctor, and I had to wait three more weeks for that. At that second appointment, a quick glance told my doctor that I had vaginal dryness from low estrogen, which would also explain why my tear was hurting as well. She gave me a prescription for vaginal cream and a few weeks later I was feeling 100 percent better.

At the same time, I was battling a urinary tract infection in addition to the vaginal dryness. I was on antibiotics for a month to combat this persistent UTI, and I felt so embarrassed to have a UTI that wouldn't go away. Apparently, low estrogen leads not only to vaginal dryness but also UTIs, so now I wonder whether, if I had fixed the estrogen problem first, I might not have been on antibiotics for so long (if at all)! The only bright spot in that story is that because I was taking probiotics, I did not develop a yeast infection with prolonged antibiotic use. Because I have long had gut problems, I have found a probiotic really can make a difference in helping digestion and fighting off bad bacteria.

The other complaint I had during that first appointment with the nurse practitioner was pain during intercourse. It had been over six months now since I gave birth, and in addition to the blisters, I just wasn't comfortable. It felt like there was a wall in the way. The nurse didn't give me any information or advice, but through my own research I did discover that there was a wall: my sagging pelvic floor.

Pelvic Floor

When I discovered that my pelvic floor was sagging, I had no idea what to do about it, or still exactly what my pelvic floor was. Now I know that the pelvic floor is a group of muscles that stretches like a hammock from the pubic bone to the tailbone. It supports a group of other muscles, including the bladder, uterus, and colon. "Think about it as a sling of muscles that your torso sits in. You don't have to be having incontinence issues to need pelvic floor strength. A weak or tight pelvic floor can cause SI joint pain, low back and hip pain."[14] It also can disrupt your sexual function.

I had heard about Kegels to strengthen your pelvic floor, but I had no idea if I was squeezing the right muscle. In *The Postnatal Depletion Cure*, Dr. Serralach says you can test the strength of your pelvic floor when you are urinating. Try to stop the flow of urine midstream. If you can't, even if it's just a small trickle, it means

---

[14] Sarah Duvall, "Trust Your Pelvic Floor Again: Strengthening Beyond Kegels," *Core Exercise Solutions*, July 29, 2019, https://coreexercisesolutions.com/articles/best-pelvic-floor-exercises/.

your pelvic floor is too weak. If you pee while jumping, running, or even sneezing, you need to strengthen your pelvic floor!

I am not a muscle expert, but from what I've learned, the abdominals, hip flexors, glutes, and pelvic floor all work in connection with one another. It's all about balance, and if one muscle is too loose or too tight, it affects all the other muscles and joints. I had a physical therapist explain to me that the pelvic floor could also be too tight or too short, and therefore a Kegel alone is not a great solution to fix your pelvic floor problem. A Kegel does not help to relax or lengthen your pelvic floor, and it doesn't work your other core muscles along with it. A full, deep squat (with your butt out) is more likely to help all those muscles work together. You can find instructions on the Internet (now that you know what you are looking for). Or better yet, make an appointment with a physical therapist to help look for muscle tightness or weakness, and the therapist can give you a personalized plan for recovery.

By strengthening your pelvic floor, you are not only helping your bladder control and sexual function (which, in turn, helps your marriage), but you are helping the other muscles in your abdomen work together to create a stronger core, which will give you the foundation for proper posture.

A weak pelvic floor is becoming a problem for more and more women because we have poor posture in general, and we often sit on soft couches and chairs that contribute to bad posture and weak abdominal muscles. Also, I was told that the pelvic floor can take up to three months to heal after delivery. In those first three months, the books I read said to be very careful about exercising so as to not strain your pelvic floor any more than it might already be. Luckily, I'm not great at exercising, so I'm pretty sure that wasn't my problem.

Exercise

"Movement is an essential part of being healthy, as it helps get blood and oxygen to your cells. Movement includes posture, core strength, alignment, and a good walking style."[15]

One time, at a birthday party, I cornered a family-practice doctor to ask her about losing the baby belly. I had learned what diastasis recti was but was looking for some advice from this doctor to heal it, since she sees a lot of postpartum women and has children herself. She was really caught off guard (perhaps because we were at a child's birthday party), but the best answer she managed to give me was that she heard that going gluten free could reduce inflammation and that, if it was really bad, there was surgery to correct it. She didn't mention any specific exercises to help strengthen the core after having a baby, as I was hoping a doctor with her experience could.

The problem for me, at five months postpartum after Zoe was born, was that I still looked as if I were five months pregnant, and my belly stuck out way past my chest. My husband pushed on my abdomen and declared he couldn't feel any muscles. I made an appointment with the chiropractor because I was having a hard time standing up straight and was having frequent hip pain. He gave me an adjustment but told me my spine was looking good. He advised me to lay off the dairy, which can cause inflammation and could be preventing me from losing belly weight.

I struggled to believe that all my belly weight was due to eating gluten or dairy, as I was eating healthier than before, yet I was still unable to lose the weight. I did decide it was time to start exercising again, so I climbed on the treadmill and was proud of myself when I walked for eight minutes straight. I was breathing

[15] Serrallach, *Postnatal Depletion Cure*, 54.

heavy and aching all over, which meant I was definitely out of shape! A few weeks later, I hit another milestone: walking on the treadmill for twelve minutes before giving up.

With previous postpartum exercises, I tried Jillian Michaels' *Six-Week Six-Pack* abs workout, complete with planks and crunches a few months after giving birth, but this time I could definitely not hold myself up. I now know that doing planks, crunches, and leg lifts right after having a baby can worsen diastasis recti instead of fixing it, especially if you don't do them properly, so it's possible I had been making the problem worse over time. For Mother's Day, my friend and I bought ourselves a subscription to an online postpartum-recovery workout program.

After putting the kids to bed one night, I logged on and watched the intro video to the program. As I sat in my office chair, I felt as if the instructor was talking directly to me. I wept as she described my struggles to reconnect with my body, find my strength, stand tall, and lose the belly. She promised results and a holistic approach that included wearing flat shoes, walking for twenty minutes every day, and eating a healthy diet.

I discovered then that I had diastasis recti and that's why my husband couldn't locate my ab muscles. They had been separated in pregnancy and were unable to return to normal on their own. I suspect that the separation became larger with each pregnancy. I also had pelvic floor issues. The abdominal core is a whole system of muscles that need to work together, and when they don't, some muscles tighten and some have too much slack (hence my hip pain). I learned the proper position to stand and sit straight, and the program emphasized the importance of squatting properly to use your core instead of your back.

As I began the program, I noticed how much squatting and bending I do on a regular basis to pick up the baby, unload the dishwasher, buckle seat belts, do laundry, and so forth. I also realized how much I slouch while nursing and while standing at the kitchen counter, which I do for hours every day. But finally learning the proper procedure helped me to practice my exercises throughout the day. For the first time in almost a year, I had hope that I had found an answer to help me reconnect with my body.

"Twenty minutes of brisk exercising five times a week is part of God's plan for the body," a wise priest once told me. I've had a bad relationship with exercise going back to middle school. As a straight-A student, the two classes I got Bs in were gym class and geometry. I was not good at sports and was always picked last to be on a team. Even in high school, I couldn't run for a whole mile without taking walking breaks to catch my breath.

The beauty of brisk exercise, though, is that it can be simply walking at a slightly quicker pace; enough to break a little sweat and get my heart racing. With only one or two babies, it was easy to put them in the stroller and go for a walk. The fresh air, sun, and change of scenery do much for the body and the soul. It got too hard with four kids and homeschooling to get regular walks in, so I bought a used treadmill on Craigslist for sixty dollars. I have tried walking early in the morning or after putting the kids to bed, but neither of those times have worked well for me. I'm not a morning person, and I'm too exhausted by the end of the day. What I enjoy is getting a break from the kids right after dinner and decompressing for twenty minutes on the treadmill. My introverted self craves that alone time, and then I can shower and be ready for bed. That time doesn't always work, though, so sometimes I have to get creative.

A couple of months after I had gotten a Fitbit watch, Nathan and I were hurriedly wrangling the kids to get dressed for Mass. As I glanced at my watch to check the time while pulling a toddler's pants on, I was surprised to see that I was in full out "fat-burning" mode. Getting all the kids out the door can be quite the workout!

Ironically, the days I usually get the most steps in are not the days I go walking on the treadmill; they are the days I do laundry or shop at Costco. I'm either running up and down the stairs with loads of laundry or pushing my heavy cart around the big-box store (not to mention putting away all the items I buy there!), and those steps add up. If you are discouraged by not finding time to work out, start with making the chores you already do work for you.

> Regular exercise improves immune function and increases the production of antioxidant substances in the body. It helps you to sleep better at night and feel more energetic during the day. A brisk walk does wonders for depression and anxiety. A bout of exercise helps to suppress your appetite for sweets and junk food and increases your appetite for natural, nourishing foods. Flexibility and muscular strength stave off uneven strain on the skeleton that can lead to pain and injury over time.[16]

The one mantra I kept hearing during my research is that it's important to start out slow and increase gradually. In fact, some women (even athletes!) do not return to prepregnancy fitness levels for up to two years. You cannot rush strengthening muscles and loosening ligaments. Some muscles tighten to try and make up for looser muscles, and if you are working out too hard, those tight muscles can cause pain and injury. I have had to build a solid foundation for correct posture, movement, and breathing

[16] Raffelock and Rountree, *Natural Guide to Pregnancy*, 243.

before I could get good exercise in, and I wouldn't even say I've done the best job.

Posture

A year later, after dabbling with exercise off and on, I still wasn't at my goal. I had gained (some) muscle and healed the diastasis recti below my belly button, but I struggled with the separation above my belly button, and I still had a lot of pounds to lose.

While my spine was technically straight according to the chiropractor, it was apparent to me that my muscles were not holding my spine up. My head tilted forward, my shoulders slouched, my neck was always tight, and this was causing a considerable amount of pain. When I complained to the chiropractor about my neck and shoulder pain, he rubbed the muscles but told me that was just my "mommy muscle" getting overused as I carried kids around. But as I began to research postpartum exercises, I discovered how important posture was and how wrong I had been standing. The reality for these aches and pains was poor posture: hunched shoulders, belly sticking out, and hips and butt tucked in.

Not only that, but my observant husband noticed that I was walking with my left foot turned in, so no wonder most of my pain was on my left side. That's when I realized that my exercise was futile if I wasn't doing it with proper posture. I wouldn't be strengthening my core while walking hunched over; instead, I would be overtaxing my back and other muscles. In addition, those with forward head posture are more likely to have pelvic floor issues![17] If I was going to reap the benefits of walking and exercise, I had to be standing properly.

[17] Duvall, "The Best Pelvic Floor Exercises."

When I began standing properly, it felt at first as if I was sticking my chest and butt out, but that was because I was used to slouching. By putting my thumbs on my ribcage and stretching my pinkies to my pelvic bone, I could make sure my ribs and pelvis were aligned over one another. This usually meant I had to push my pelvis back (which felt to me like sticking my butt out) to give my spine the natural curve it's meant to have.

Your core should be holding you up, your shoulders should be relaxed, your glutes shouldn't be clenched, and your weight should be distributed evenly between the ball and the heel of each foot, with toes spread slightly (which is why wearing flat shoes is good for practicing posture).

My hamstrings were too tight as well, so I had to begin stretching my legs and hips every day in order to stand properly, as well as remind myself dozens of times over the course of the day to correct my posture. Thankfully, the stretches and reminders did make a difference, and my aches and pains began to disappear. As another bonus, good posture helped me to breathe correctly. The difference between a deep breath and a shallow breath is a big one!

Breathing

"Take a deep breath," the lady on the video told me. "Do your shoulders rise up? Does your belly stick out? If your shoulders are rising up and your belly is not extending out, you are breathing too shallow. Shallow, chest-breathing does not give you the oxygen and relaxation that deep, belly breathing does."

Apparently, correct breathing can be the difference between a strong, pain-free body and one that's under constant cortisol distress, which leads to anxiety and inflammation. When you breathe, your shoulders shouldn't move much, but your chest and your belly should: they should expand as your diaphragm contracts to stimulate your vagus nerve, telling your brain to relax. Relaxation helps with digestion, sleep, sex, and that good ol' number two. If you let only your belly expand, you are not contracting your diaphragm. Too much belly movement can also put unnecessary strain on muscles that could be trying to heal, such as a diastasis recti.

"As you inhale, your belly should rise. At the same time, you should feel your lower ribs and back expand, almost like a round cylinder. Ideally, your shoulders remain relaxed. The last place to move is your upper chest," writes Dr. Serrallach.[18] Breathe through your nose. Let your ribcage expand in all directions. Breathe slowly: count to four as you breathe in, and to seven as you breathe out.

Now I was starting to feel a little overwhelmed about how I would remember not only to stand and walk properly, but now how to breathe properly too! Luckily, the more I practiced, the easier it became. I still find that if I have gone a few months without much exercise or stretching, my breathing is poorer and my muscles are stiffer. So, it seems that every few months I have to return to being intentional about my exercise, posture, and breathing.

Sleep

Sleep is the killer. Every postpartum mom needs sleep, but it can be so hard to come by. For their first few months, my babies usually slept in our Fisher-Price swing. The cushy sides and cradle

---

[18] Serrallach, *Postnatal Depletion Cure*, 117.

shape of the swing provided an environment to help them get to sleep. I could never get them to sleep in a crib until about four or five months, when they were rolling around and had grown out of the swing. Also, my husband is a light sleeper and barely got a wink of sleep if the baby was in the same room. So the swing was a win-win-win because the baby stayed asleep longer, which meant I got more sleep, and so did my husband. I felt guilty about this sleeping arrangement at first, until someone told me it was okay, and that her baby also slept in a swing. I was afraid that my babies wouldn't transition well to a crib, but when they were ready, it wasn't a problem. The most important thing, other than safety, is that everyone is getting enough sleep!

Marilyn Shannon says:

> I am convinced that many women do not recognize their own symptoms of chronic sleep deprivation because it is so much a part of their lives. I think many just consider themselves as having low energy, or being stressed or irritable by temperament, when lack of sleep is actually the underlying cause of these symptoms.... You will feel better, think better, look better, and enjoy life more if you go through it in a rested state. You will be more cheerful. You will manage stress better. Your immune system will work better. And you will be more productive if you spend the time you need sleeping, because it will increase your energy and mental focus during your waking time.[19]

I have always been a good sleeper. I usually don't have a problem getting to sleep, but it's not getting *enough* sleep that hits me hard. I need about eight hours of sleep to function like a normal

[19] Shannon, *Fertility, Cycles, and Nutrition*, 58.

person. So, I had to strategize ways to get the sleep I needed. For one, it meant filling my babies up with milk and getting them to sleep for four- to five-hour stretches early on. I would take a long time to nurse them in the middle of the night, being up for about an hour, so I could get another four- to five-hour stretch. It also meant taking a nap when my husband came home from work, or sleeping in and letting my husband handle the morning routine. It meant sleeping when the baby slept and putting a movie on for the other kids. I think it's one reason why the early months after Zoe's arrival were the easiest out of all four kids: I had finally learned the value of sleep (and vitamins).

When I ask moms what they would do differently the next time they are postpartum, many of them say that they would get more sleep. That might mean sleeping when the baby is sleeping, or having someone watch the baby so Mom can get a nap in, and using whatever it takes to get that baby to sleep! It's that important!

Consider these effects of sleep deprivation:[20]
- difficulty in finding the words to finish sentences
- struggling with decision-making
- inability to multitask
- craving junk food
- weakened immune system

Here are some tools to help you get to sleep:
- lavender essential oil in a diffuser
- blackout curtains or an eye mask, or both
- avoiding screens before bed
- drinking hot herbal tea before bed

[20] Serrallach, *Postnatal Depletion Cure*, 33–34.

- avoiding carbs or sugar, or drinking too much water, before bed
- eating a small, protein-based snack before bed
- breathing and stretching as part of your bedtime routine

A small amount of melatonin before bed can be helpful, but talk to your health practitioner before taking it.

Bringing It All Together

Overall, my postpartum journey has forced me to recognize the importance of taking care of my body as the visible expression of my soul. Grace builds upon nature, but I never understood what that meant until I had kids. When I get more sleep, keep up my vitamin levels, and give my body exercise, I am more disposed to receive God's grace to be present to my family and to love my spouse. By taking care of my body, I am glorifying God through being better able to live out my vocation as a wife and a mother.

On the other hand, when my body is not working as God intended, because I'm binging on chocolate, not exercising, and not taking naps when I need them, it's hard for me to think straight, get up in the morning, and love my family. And the more overwhelmed I feel by life, the less likely I am to pray. I end up watching TV and ignoring the more pressing matters in life because it all feels too hard. Simple things such as vitamins, sleep, and exercise make a big difference, not only in my relationship with God but in my marriage as well.

5

Marriage and NFP

Practicing NFP during postpartum is the worst. Your fertility markers are all over the place, and you never quite know when you will be fertile again. Waking up multiple times during the night may mean you didn't allow enough hours to go by to pee on a stick, or consecutive hours of sleep to get an accurate temperature reading—not to mention that your libido is usually at an all-time low. So it's no wonder that postpartum hits your marriage like a hurricane and spins your relationship into a vortex of chaos and a deluge of tears.

I can see the temptation to use contraception. I've heard many Catholics try to argue this point: with PPD, emotional adjustments, physical recovery, the expense of having a baby, and highly irregular fertility markers, contraception can be justified after having a baby. The nurses at the hospital will even push it on you only hours after you've pushed your baby out. So, it seems like a good idea to use contraception, have sex whenever you want, and not think about a baby for a while. Well, it seems like a good idea at first.

I've been searching the Bible to try to find somewhere that Jesus says, "Forgive me for making discipleship so difficult at times. Let me make an exception because I definitely don't want you to suffer any more than you already have." Only, I can't find that verse (but believe me, I've looked!). I've heard women say, "Have to struggle with NFP? That's not the God of love I know." Yet I have to respond, " 'Willing to make exceptions for difficulties' is not the God of love I know." And that's because now I truly believe that the suffering that comes from being faithful to NFP in your marriage after having a baby is the stuff that saints are made of.

I love my children, and even though Lily screamed bloody murder every time I changed her diaper, I still changed it. She hated it, but it was good for her. I absolutely hate practicing NFP postpartum, and I'm usually not good at it (which is why most of my children are less than two years apart). But God asks me to do difficult things because, in the end, it's good for me. Practice makes perfect, so now, eight years into marriage, my husband and I are getting better at using NFP for spacing, and my children are close in age and therefore have the best playmates. I have no regrets now about having our children when we did, although I may have had some at the time.

I remember yelling at my mom, who has been teaching and promoting NFP since before I was born. I told her they lied: NFP wasn't happy or fun or good for our marriage. We were not financially stable. I was not emotionally stable. And we were having kids faster than I could keep up with. I felt as if Nathan and I were on different planets, and more than pulling us closer, the unknowns and waiting periods of NFP seemed to be causing resentment and pushing us further away from each other.

That was three years into our marriage, and what really helped us was to activate the grace of the sacrament of Matrimony. We had said "for better or worse," and now we needed God to help us stick it out. We were faithful to using NFP, and so the benefits eventually came, but we had to work through all the hard stuff to get to the payoff. What I've come to understand is that NFP is good for marriage in the long run; it's not a short-term gain.

We've also learned so much along the way that has made our marriage stronger. On a retreat, a priest described the process of forging a knife: heating and pounding the metal, cooling it, heating it again, honing it against a stone. But how he summarized the process is what struck me: The blacksmith is not trying to hurt the knife; he's trying to perfect it. God, who is all good, would never want to *hurt* us, but He does want to *perfect* us. When God allows us to go through trials in our marriage, it is because, in His infinite wisdom, He knows it can ultimately bring about good in us, provided we accept His grace.

A girlfriend asked me once how long it took before my husband and I started to get on the same page about parenting and NFP. I told her eight years and four kids. Everything before that was pretty hard. There were even some really bad times in those eight years when I questioned my love for Nathan and why I married him in the first place. There were times when we stormed out on each other and gave each other the cold shoulder. I'm not proud of those moments, but it's how we ultimately responded to them that made the difference: we went back to our marital promises. We had entered into a covenant that could not be broken, so now we had to figure it out. And our love now is stronger precisely *because* of the difficulties rather than *in spite of them*. If we had had it easy and never fought or struggled to love each other, there would be no refinement.

The grace of the sacrament of Matrimony is real and effective, provided we are disposed to receive it. Christ, who has shown His love for us on the Cross, "encounters Christian spouses through the sacrament of Matrimony."[21] Grace is the gift by which Christ enters into us and transforms our ability to love. The *Catechism of the Catholic Church* beautifully says that through Matrimony, "Christ dwells with them [spouses], gives them the strength to take up their crosses and so follow him, to rise again after they have fallen, to forgive one another, to bear one another's burdens ... and to love one another with supernatural, tender, fruitful love."[22]

I've seen very clearly through these postpartum times in our marriage that I need God's grace to love my husband, to practice NFP, and to raise our children. I can't do it without Christ, because I don't have that supernatural love on my own. I'm sure our marriage will have other tough times ahead, but because we have navigated four postpartum periods, I feel hopeful that, with the help of God's grace, we can navigate whatever other difficulties come our way.

Another benefit of using NFP came with having to respect the natural cycle of fertility and work with it, instead of against it. One surprising thing about fertility, even when we are abstaining, is that it reminds us that we still like each other after all these kids and all these years. It's refreshing to know that even with my saggy skin (from being pregnant four times), my husband is still attracted to me. We can still flirt, and anticipating phase-3 infertility gives us something to look forward to. This cycle of fertility and abstaining has definitely given us relational rough patches, but over the years, it has ultimately kept our love alive and exciting.

Practicing abstinence before marriage and NFP during marriage has also forced us to find other ways to love each other. I

---

[21] *Catechism of the Catholic Church* (CCC), no. 1642.
[22] Ibid.

had no idea how much this would benefit our marriage postpartum, because there is not very much lovemaking in the months after having a baby. Since we had practiced abstinence before, we knew we could do it again while I recovered from delivery and again when we were unsure of our returning fertility. I look back in gratitude for being able to navigate that, because I see other couples who don't know how to express their love for their spouses in other ways, and they grow distant.

It's also important to recognize that men struggle with the transition to parenthood as well and with the periods of abstinence that likely follow. They have not gone through the bodily changes and hormone shifts that we have, and try as they might, I just don't think they can quite understand. In addition, they are used to having all the love and attention of their spouses, and now they have to share it with the baby. They may feel guilty for feeling that way, but it's an adjustment for them to have a new member of the family, just as it is for us mothers. Dads also struggle with sleep deprivation and depression, so we can't shut them out. It's hard to talk about all the changes taking place, but we need to be able to go through this transition together. We need to be able to be vulnerable with one another.

NFP: The Methods and the Madness

My husband and I took a Couple to Couple League (CCL) Sympto-Thermal class when we were engaged. We listened along and charted but never took it seriously, apparently, because Timothy was a honeymoon baby. I didn't really think twice about looking into any other methods because my parents had been teaching for CCL for as long as I've been alive.

Sympto-Thermal means you are charting your mucus signs and your basal body temperature for signs of fertility and then using formulas to determine fertile or infertile windows of time (i.e., the likelihood of conceiving a baby). You can also check your cervix, but I don't.

After Lily was born, we were not ready to have another child, and I was so nervous about charting. So, for Christmas, my mother got us the Clearblue fertility monitor, which uses your first urine sample of the day to determine fertility levels. Now with checking urine, mucus, and temperature, I became a lot more confident with charting. When I got pregnant with Luke, it was because of stress-delayed ovulation (which, by the way, is a real thing), and apparently was all part of God's plan for us.

After Zoe was born, my husband and I decided we needed an NFP refresher, so we took a self-paced postpartum course online through CCL. We used the Clearblue monitor in addition to charting, which helped to mark a few months of infertility, but then for a few months it still meant a lot of uncertainty and abstinence.

Thanks to my high-potency vitamins' boosting my hormone function, when my fertility returned I was able to become more confident in my cycle than I ever had before. Usually after my fertility returns postpartum, my cycles are forty to fifty days long with signs all over the place. This time around, my cycles became very regular almost immediately (twenty-eight to thirty-one days), and the signs were more obvious.

I know a lot of couples who use Creighton, especially if they are struggling with infertility or subfertility, but I don't know a lot about that method, except that it also checks for mucus and has fun baby stickers. The good news is that fertility awareness methods (FAMs) are becoming more popular, and there are a lot of apps that can help you chart, provided you have the knowledge of how your fertility works.

No matter what method of natural family planning you use, I recommend finding some support so you aren't walking this journey alone. I like the quarterly magazine *Family Foundations* for anyone who needs some encouragement in going against the tide. The magazine is put out by the Couple to Couple League, an organization that has been around for about fifty years, long before "natural" was popular. In the last few years, their magazine has touched on a lot of really relevant topics, such as postpartum NFP, stay-at-home moms versus working moms, parenting using Theology of the Body concepts, NFP from a dad's point of view, irregular cycles, and a whole lot more.

Another resource that I like is naturalwomanhood.org, whose goal is to help women understand their bodies and improve their health through fertility charting and natural methods. There's also a newer online community called Off the Charts that provides support, education, and connection for those who want to practice the NFP lifestyle better. You can find out more by visiting www.offthechartsnfp.com.

Lastly, make sure you have a friend or two whom you can talk to! Nothing can replace the personal relationship and encouragement that comes from a friend walking the same road as you.

Intimacy

While I was pregnant with Zoe, I would cry just thinking about being postpartum: the sleepless nights, the stubborn weight, the leaky boobs, the fights with my husband. Lack of sleep makes us both a little cranky, and my depression and wild hormones make for an even bumpier ride. I've torn with each delivery, and the stitches take the longest to heal. Add to that vaginal dryness from breastfeeding, and sex with my husband is the very last thing I want, ever. Bowls of ice cream and Netflix? Yes. Being intimate in the place where a baby pushed his way out into the world only two months earlier? Not so much.

You'd think that we were lovemaking fiends with how quickly I would get pregnant again, but it just turned out that those few and far-between times were the fertile ones.

The good news is that with each baby, we've been able to learn from the one before. I need *more* than the requisite six weeks before resuming intercourse; that's a given. I need to ease my way into it. I need estrogen cream. And I definitely need to strengthen my pelvic floor!

It would be easy (for me!) to say, "I just had a baby; let's take a year off from intercourse." Now, a couple might discern very valid reasons for doing so, but the majority of couples like us just need to work together to find some balance. The way I thought about it was this: Intimacy should have a place of primacy in your married life, because it is the very thing that made you married in the first place. Sexual union completes the sacrament of Matrimony as two become one flesh. Therefore, every time you engage in the marital embrace, you are renewing the promises you made on your wedding day, as well as inviting grace into your marriage to help you love one another.

Still, sometimes I have to "fake it 'til I make it" until around nine months postpartum, and now my husband knows that the times before then will be less often. In addition, we have to start charting again, and it's always scary when you don't know when your fertility will return. It's like slowly turning the handle on a jack-in-the-box, waiting for the flashing ovulation sign on your monitor to pop up and say, "Surprise"!

In a Facebook group of Catholic women, a fellow mom reached out to say that she was struggling with making intimacy with her husband a priority. At first, she thought it was simply not wanting to get pregnant again, but lack of libido had a lot to do with it. Even with open communication and a patient husband, it was weighing on their marriage.

Let's face it, your body is just tired: tired from being pregnant, giving birth, nursing or feeding in the middle of the night. You are constantly giving of yourself! By the end of the day, you feel you have nothing left to give your husband. And if you are nursing and being touched out all day, the last thing you want is more physical touch! Also, leaky boobs are a real issue.

Once someone had the courage to admit it, other moms chimed in with the same struggle. They also had some great suggestions to make the intimacy part of marriage stronger after having a baby. Here are some of them:

- There are seasons of intimacy, and early postpartum is just one of those times where you come together less. Just remember, the season doesn't last.
- If you are a planner, secretly "schedule" having sex so it's on your list. That will keep you from moving it to the back burner.
- Mentally prepare. Have a glass of wine. Make it seem spontaneous to him even if you were secretly planning it all day.
- Try to take a nap earlier in the day, or switch it up to afternoons on the weekends.
- You might need alone time to rest and recharge. Find a hobby; get out of the house for a bit; have some quiet time.

- Have your husband help with the chores. If he knew that doing the dishes would make you more available, I'm pretty sure he would do the dishes.
- Take the pressure and expectation off by trying to remember things you did before you were married. It could be cooking together, game nights, crafting, and so forth.
- If you are nursing, do a little extra pumping or a bottle feed, if you can, so you don't feel as "touched out" by the end of the day.
- Consider at-home spa dates. Light candles; put on some background music; include massage, facials, diffusing essential oils, foot soaking and rubs, and so forth. It helps to feel intimate and sexy and might help put you in the mood.
- Beg God for the grace to help you love your husband physically and intimately!
- Check your vitamin levels. Low levels of DHEA and testosterone have a lot to do with lack of libido, along with low magnesium or essential fatty acids.
- If it hurts, get some help.

This last one is where I found myself after having Zoe. Our intimacy was dampened by my fear, my pain, and my unwillingness to talk about it or try to work it out. I felt the weight of being a disappointment, even though my husband was so patient and gracious about it. But he also was encouraging me by this point to go get checked out. That's partly how I ended up on the exam table with the nurse practitioner examining my vaginal ring of blisters.

The help of estrogen cream and the exercises to strengthen my pelvic floor made all the difference in our marriage. Our intimacy began to flourish because I finally got the help I needed.

This time of troubleshooting also forced us to talk about our sex life more. I needed to have my love tank filled before feeling able to be intimate. My primary love language is quality time; thus, I had to feel that we were connecting on an emotional level before we could connect on a physical level. We could straighten up the house together, watch a show, cuddle on the couch, or share about our dreams and disappointments. Once that happened, I was in a better place to receive him.

I also know that I need a lot of sleep, and being tired causes me to shut down. There are definitely times when I am so exhausted and touched out that no amount of quality time will help—only sleep. My husband now understands that this isn't a rejection of him, but a physical fact. I have been better able to verbalize my needs and let him know when I need a nap after dinner or to sleep in on the weekend if he wants me to be more physically available.

Focusing on Marriage

When my parents would come out to visit after I had a baby, they would encourage Nathan and me to go out by ourselves after dinner. Often we were so tired that we would have rather just gone to bed, but we didn't want to waste the opportunity. We usually found ourselves wandering around Home Depot for a half hour, then ending up at Village Inn for pie. It was the lamest of dates, but at this exhausted phase in our life, it was the best we could manage.

Babies are very needy (as are toddlers), so it was sometimes hard to put my spouse first! My babies demanded much of my time and energy, and it was easy to feel resentful that my husband wanted my time and energy, too. A friend reminded me, though, that *marriage*, not motherhood, is the sacrament. Quality time with my husband doesn't just magically happen, so I learned that I needed to be intentional about it. "Great," I thought. "One last thing to try to be intentional about and fail at, right?" But the good news is that putting your husband first doesn't have to be complicated or time-consuming. This is where the simple things are the most effective. Here are some of the best suggestions I've heard:

- Hold hands when you walk. You will undoubtedly be walking somewhere together, so just reach out your hand.
- It's also a given that you will shower (every now and then). Shower together and talk about your day. It doesn't *have* to lead to anything, but it can be an intimate time anyway.
- Give each other back rubs and massages.
- Send texts letting your husband know that you are thinking about him. Leave a love note around.
- Make your husband's lunch, or do some other act of service.
- Have date night in. When the baby is sleeping, do something together! Since my husband is a woodworker and remodeler, we spent a lot of quality time dreaming and designing our next home makeover or piece of furniture. We would lie in bed after the kids were asleep and scour the Internet for inspiration, argue over the details, and eventually watch it come to life.
- Have conversations about something other than your baby. It's dangerous to be so consumed with parenthood that you can't find anything else to talk about.
- Every so often, though, we like to go through the pictures and videos we took of the kids over the last several

months. Perspective is a great reminder of the fun we have had and how far we've come. Babies change so much in their first year; we can look at pictures from a month ago and see how much our kids have grown!

• If you can, even once a month, get out of the house together. It could be a traditional dinner date or more of a hobby-oriented date. Last year, for our anniversary, Nathan and I took a glass-blowing class together, and it was a blast!

I've heard the saying "A good babysitter is cheaper than marriage counseling." The thought behind that phrase is that it's better to be proactive than to put out fires, which is true. And yet, it's okay to go to counseling. In fact, it's a *good* thing to go to counseling. Considering the dysfunctional world we live in, I think we all need counseling at one point or another in our lives. Going to marriage counseling means that you want your marriage to be better. No one can fault you for that! Perhaps you have family nearby that can watch the kids, or perhaps you can exchange babysitting with family friends: they watch your kids, and then you watch theirs. Heck, if you live in Denver, I'll watch your kids because I believe counseling can make all the difference in a marriage.

Verbalizing Needs

One technique that really helped our marriage was when I learned to verbalize my needs with my husband. I know he's not a mind reader, but I just kind of hoped he'd see my exasperation and look for ways to help. Since it didn't work out that way, I learned to be more specific with what I needed. Otherwise my exasperation would lead to an explosion with yelling or tears because I let the emotion build up. Then Nathan would ask why I didn't just let him know how I was feeling sooner. I would reply that it didn't occur to me to do so until I exploded, so I realized I needed to be more conscious of how I was feeling and to express that.

I began to tell Nathan very specifically, "I'm not going to make it until bedtime, so I need to lie down for a bit after dinner. Can you clean up the dishes while I nap?" Or I would suggest that if he could clear the table and wipe it down while I did the dishes, we could have more time together in the evening. Also, since I'm incredibly introverted, I would sometimes tell him that I just needed some alone time. Often after a baby was born, I'd go grocery shopping at 8:00 p.m. and wander the aisles by myself as a way to unwind while getting something done.

While I became more adept at verbalizing my needs, I also needed to become more aware of my husband's needs. He needed me to be present to him. He needed time to play cards with his buddies or snowboard in the winter. He needed some downtime after work to relax, too. He also needed me to step back and let him grow in fatherhood by allowing him to care for our babies in his own way.

In some studies, fathers who hold their babies in those first few weeks after birth have shown a decrease in testosterone and an increase in prolactin. This hormone can help them to feel not only more bonded with their babies but more sensitive to the babies' needs. I find that my husband doesn't ask to hold the baby often, but if I ask him to, he is happy to do it. So I made a conscious effort to give him the baby when he was around so he would get that bonding time in. I would also specifically ask for help with changing clothes and diapers and bathing, because again, he wouldn't always offer, but he'd take on the task when asked!

Dr. Oscar Serrallach confirmed my findings when he wrote, "Women often don't realize that most men really do want to contribute and play an active role in raising the baby, but they are better able to help when they feel they have specific tasks or duties that belong to them. You want to make him feel not only that you are honoring his contribution but that this will in turn satisfy your needs as a mother and partner.... They want to provide solutions!"[23]

Fathers interact with kids differently than mothers do, and that's okay. Just because I do something one way doesn't mean Nathan has to do it the same way. We each have a different routine for Zoe when we put her to bed, but both routines have the same end result: she goes to sleep. Let dads have the freedom to make their own connections and do things differently than you do, as long as you are unified in the important things. I learned the hard way not to hover and express my opinions on Nathan's style of play! He is much more fun than I am when it comes to playtime, anyway.

The bottom line is that in order to grow as a family, I have to stay connected with my spouse. When you are each busy with your responsibilities, it's easy to get isolated. In addition, small problems we had before having a baby became larger problems after birth — communication styles, arguments, finances, hobbies, and so forth. We were forced to work on solving these problems while admitting our weaknesses along the way. It isn't easy to share your vulnerabilities, even with your spouse, but it's the only way to move forward. We have had to say "I'm sorry" and "I forgive you" repeatedly, but we are definitely growing in patience and humility!

[23] Serrallach, *Postnatal Depletion Cure*, 248.

6

Mental Health

I have never been good at multitasking. On the one hand, it makes me a great friend since I can be fully present to a conversation. On the other hand, it makes it difficult to have a conversation with a friend at the park while trying to keep an eye on my kids, or even to nurse a baby while talking to my older kids. I can't cook a meal and help keep my toddler busy at the same time. It has taken me years to be able to clean the house while listening to a podcast!

Postpartum is simply a difficult time for my mental health. I don't do well without getting seven and a half hours of uninterrupted sleep. I am also prone to anxiety and am sensitive to loud noises. When there is too much commotion going on, I shut down or completely lose it. There will be screaming babies, milk on the floor, dirty dishes in the sink, and I just can't handle it.

After a year of working on my health goals after Zoe was born, I landed in the doctor's office for anxiety again. I was taking plenty of vitamins, was exercising occasionally; and was in a good place in my marriage. But my temper was on a short fuse, and on several occasions, I had almost gone hoarse from yelling. My brain was foggy, and I had troubling remembering to-do lists and bill schedules. My social anxiety kept me from leaving the house or responding to texts. I would lie awake at night, exhausted, and yet my brain wouldn't stop analyzing an earlier conversation a million times over.

One day, as I was about to lose it on my children again, I saw the look of fear in their eyes, and it struck me in the heart. My children were afraid of me. I had tried everything in my power to control my temper and yet still failed so completely and miserably that I knew I needed help.

At my OB/GYN's office, I explained to the nurse practitioner that I was doing fine right after Zoe was born, but I knew I wasn't myself anymore. My NFP charts no longer showed a basic infertile pattern, and my body was shifting gears to return to fertility, although it would take a few more months for it finally to return. The nurse told me she was proud of me for coming to get help. She was proud of the steps I had taken to exercise and supplement with vitamins. I had a good support system with my husband and my moms' group, and my parents were moving to town after my dad's retirement. So she offered me Zoloft and told me that it was safe to take while breastfeeding and had few side effects. I hated the idea of going on medication, but I was desperate.

Thankfully, the Zoloft worked, and my only regret was not having taken it sooner. Somehow, I felt calmer and could think more clearly. I no longer had a raging anger burning inside me at all times. My social anxiety decreased (but did not entirely disappear). I answered text messages.

Still, medicine didn't solve all my problems; it just helped me to be able to manage them. I now had a choice again. I had developed some good habits along the way, but I had some bad coping habits as well. And I still struggle with choosing joy and not losing my temper.

I finally weaned myself off Zoloft after a little over a year. I had made great strides on the medicine, but I wanted to try to get off it. I was okay with a lower dose, but when I tried to go off it completely, I didn't do so well. So, I kept a lower dose while supplementing with Ashwagandha root, which is an herb powder proven to lower cortisol, combat anxiety and depression, and reduce blood sugar levels, among other benefits. Also, it has none of the side effects that other medicines have, such as fatigue and weight gain with Zoloft. After a while, I was able to go off both, right around the time I started on thyroid medication.

Whatever it was, I felt as if I was relying on *something* to make me feel more normal. I don't handle the postpartum time well, and I have often felt embarrassed that I struggle so much to adjust to new phases of motherhood. Shouldn't this all come a little more naturally? When it doesn't, I feel like a failure.

Negative Self-Talk

A speaker at a retreat I went to said a phrase that has stuck with me ever since: "The devil condemns, but the Spirit convicts." Over the next few weeks, I became more aware of the voices that I was hearing in my head. I began to recognize a steady stream of accusations such as: "You can't even get the dishes done before bed. You are such a failure." Or, "You can never be on time for park dates and meetings. You just shouldn't go anywhere if you are always going to be late. No one is going to want to be your friend."

At this time, I was going to a mom's Rosary group on the other side of town. It started at 9:30 a.m. with the Rosary, and I almost always came in on the last decade. I was really wrestling with the voice in my head telling me not to go because I always miss the prayers, but I wanted to fight it. I wanted to prove to myself that I *can* be on time for once. Wednesday morning came, and I got up early to eat and get dressed and be ready to go. Only, the kids slept in late and wouldn't cooperate with getting dressed. The baby nursed extra long and then pooped out of her outfit minutes before we were to leave. After I finally had everyone buckled in the car and was only running a few minutes behind, I looked for my keys. They were nowhere to be found. I searched the diaper bag, my purse, and every flat surface in the house. I yelled at the kids, demanding that they tell me where they put my keys. "Maybe in the laundry room?" "I think they are in Daddy's shop." "I put them in the bathroom."

They clearly had no clue where my keys were, and now I was going to be *really* late. After sending out a desperate plea to St. Anthony, I found the keys hidden under toys on the basement floor. The Rosary was over, but I decided that since the kids were already buckled (albeit angry for being stuck in their seats for so long), we would still go, and I would make the walk of shame to the back of the room for being late. The whole twenty-minute drive there, I attacked myself for not putting my keys away, for not noticing that the toddler had taken them, and for not being on time. I chided myself for my inevitable failures because, well, that's who I am: a failure.

By now, I pretty much had my seat secured in the back of the room by the exit door. Every so often, someone other than I would come slinking in that exit door to avoid the front of the room. It was locked from the outside, and I'd usually be the one to open it. This particular morning, after finding the lost keys and coming in well after the Rosary, someone knocked at the exit door, and I let her in. A comment was made about how I was always the one to open the back door, and I replied that it was because I was perpetually late. She replied back, "Well, there are some saints who were doorkeepers."

Padre Pio, André Bessette, Solanus Casey: all were doormen. All used that role as their path to sainthood. As I mulled that over in my heart, I realized how I let the devil condemn me instead of offering up those struggles. I was embarrassed about my post as doorwoman because it was a sign of my tardiness, yet God can use even those moments to make me a saint, if I let Him. As I read up on the lives of St. André Bessette and Bl. Solanus Casey, the simple doormen who worked miracles, I knew that the only way to battle Satan's tormenting taunts was to turn to Jesus and offer up the little things to Him. So I began to offer Him my lateness, my mental anxiety, my weakness. Over time, I saw a change in my attitude and my relationship with God. Although my lateness and anxiety never fully disappeared, they didn't discourage me the way they used to.

What I've come to learn is that negative self-talk is from the devil. Jesus is firm and truthful, but not harsh and accusing. During a talk I heard on a retreat, the speaker, Fr. Riley, said we must confess negative self-talk to be freed from its grip. Another idea of his was to wear a holy medal or carry a rosary on your person. As soon as you recognize a negative, condemning thought about yourself, don't entertain it! Simply reach for your rosary or medal. That act alone can help you to choose the good.

Body Image

I'm not quite five foot two, and all my life I took it for granted that I was small and thin without even trying. Exercise was never my thing, but cookies were; and growing up, it didn't make a difference in my weight. Now I look back on my thin little frame with jealousy, because it's apparent that I will never look like that again. I was able to lose some weight after Timothy was born, but then I got pregnant again. After Lily was born, I was determined to lose the weight and was able to do so just in time to get pregnant with Luke. But after Luke and Zoe were born, the weight wasn't coming off even though I was exercising more and eating better.

It has been hard not to resent motherhood for changing my body so drastically. My husband says he likes my curves, and I know my children think I'm beautiful, but it's hard for me to agree with them when I look in the mirror. I focus on my imperfections and flaws, and the huge belly that hasn't gone away. Even though my friends still treat me the same, sometimes my negative self-image has contributed to such social anxiety that I don't want to leave the house.

I want to tell myself that it doesn't matter. I ask God to help me to see myself the way He sees me, or the way my husband sees me, but it's hard. And now, two years postpartum, it's even harder, because I don't have the excuse of having just had a baby. I know that I would never treat someone differently for having extra weight, and I am always drawn to seeing the beauty in other women, but I can never seem to find the beauty in myself. As a single young adult, I didn't struggle with body image the way I do now. I thought these things were supposed to resolve themselves when you got older, but for me the opposite is true: I struggle more now.

With my latest battle of self-loathing, I was praying to God to show me how *He* sees me. What I saw was a picture of my insides, with a gnarly branch wrapped tightly around my spine. I recognized this branch as the lie of the devil that I will never be pretty enough, good enough, or thin enough. It's been growing hidden there for a while, ever so slowly squeezing me tighter and tighter as I have allowed the lie to take hold in my thoughts.

Now that I'm aware of that ugly branch, I am working, with God's help, to undo it. I brought the thoughts and images to my spiritual director, and he counseled me through it. Then he heard my confession, and as I brought it to the light, I sobbed as I received absolution and invited grace to take the place of that lie. The effects of that Confession began the healing process, but I recognize that it's going to take time and more grace to rid myself totally of the habits of negativity.

I have to remind myself that it's not about the number on the scale; it's about my attitude. It's about ordering my health toward virtue and uniting my body and soul in the way God designed. The goal is being in right relationship with my body—not worshipping it *or* degrading it.

Another thought I had was this: no record of the saints includes a description of how much they weighed throughout their lives. Your weight does not determine your level of sanctity. My pursuit of good physical health is for the end goal of being a better mom and wife, not for the sake of being fit or outwardly attractive. If I keep my priorities in check, my body should help me to attain virtue and reveal my inner self, not discourage me from being who I am meant to be.

"Man looks on the outward appearance, but the LORD looks on the heart" (1 Sam. 16:7).

The "Perfect" Mom

Just after Zoe turned one, I was at a women's prayer group, and we were talking about house cleaning. The majority of moms there shared how they were very type-A and couldn't go to bed with dishes in the sink. I was silent for most of that meeting and then went home and sobbed tears of shame and embarrassment for regularly leaving dirty dishes in the sink overnight. It was such a low point for me, because the one thing that I should have been doing right—being a stay-at-home mom—was the one thing I was failing at miserably. I was so darn tired after getting the kids in bed that dishes were often done in the morning, and the house was not being cleaned on a regular loop schedule. Granted, I was working a part-time job from home while homeschooling, and granted, the house probably wasn't as messy to some as it was to me, but compared with those moms sharing in that moms' group, I was a failure.

If I ask myself what the perfect mom looks like, I imagine she gets up before her kids to have coffee and quiet prayer time. She doesn't get frazzled with everyone's breakfast requests, and after eating, her kids all help clean up the kitchen, get dressed, and start their day. When it comes to discipline, she is firm and gentle, and when she comes up against a difficult child, she has a wise strategy for how to overcome the problem. She gets her kids to do their chores without complaining, they never watch TV, and they often go to one of their many friends' houses for dinner, because everyone loves them. When she does cook dinner, it's delicious and all her children enjoy eating it. She always makes time to work out and looks stylish whenever she leaves the house. She serves her husband selflessly, and her house is always clean.

And then there's me: I never wake up early, I'm always frazzled, my kids watch TV, and I struggle to get them to do their chores. My prayer life is scattered, and so are the toys. I stay up too late at night and still don't find time to work out regularly.

What God has been slowly revealing to me is that (A) the perfect mom doesn't exist and (B) He's not asking me to have it together or to look like every other mom. He expects me to be a work in progress. The perfection of motherhood doesn't come in the exterior actions of a clean house and of having it all together, but in the interior responses to daily chaos.

If there's one thing God doesn't mind, it's chaos. Just open the Bible to any page! Salvation history is nothing but God showing up in the midst of chaos. And in the life of Mary, it was no different. His angel announced to this unmarried teenage girl that she would be the mother of the Savior. She gave birth far from home, in a cave. She had to flee to a foreign country to save her Son's life, only to watch Him die a brutal death when He was only thirty-three. So, it's not about the external circumstances of our lives but about how we respond to them in our hearts—how we use these opportunities to grow in virtue.

I've had to tell myself over and over again that in the year or so of postpartum, it's okay to have lower expectations and to admit that you are in survival mode. I guess some moms keep it together just fine during this time, but I couldn't; and I had to acknowledge that this time didn't have to define the rest of my motherhood, and it certainly didn't mean I was a failure.

The marks of a successful mother are not that she built up her children's college fund, potty-trained them in a day, or kept the house perpetually clean. Successful motherhood looks like blowout diapers at a dinner party, spilled milk on the floor, and marker on the walls. Well, to be more specific, it looks like the way we react to those situations: seeing them as opportunities to grow in virtues such as patience, charity, temperance, and of course, humility.

The most important question I can ask myself is: *What does God think of my motherhood?* The voice of the devil condemns, but the Spirit convicts. The Father loves me more than I could ever love my children, and He knows my strengths and weaknesses. God will call me on to greater holiness because He has my best interests in mind, but He is loving and merciful about it.

Self-care

"It is easier to be an unsupported martyr than it is to be a self-caring mother."[24]

After Timothy was born, it was hard to find time to shower. I had ill-fitting clothes for my new body type, and I hated the outfits I wore. I went to a secondhand store and bought some clothes that fit better but still were not flattering or fashionable. I disliked my new-to-me clothes but told myself they were temporary. Then I got pregnant again.

I've finally had to admit that my body shape isn't going to be what it used to be. I still shop at thrift stores, but I choose clothes that I want to wear, and most people can't tell they are secondhand. I got rid of the pre-baby clothes I was holding on to in hopes of wearing again someday, but now, so many years later, they aren't trendy anymore anyway. It was a big moment for me to change my entire wardrobe, as if I were turning over a new chapter in the story of my life—one of acceptance.

I don't wear makeup every day, but when I do, it's simple and takes only two minutes to put on. There have been times when we barely left the house for weeks because of cold weather or sickness, and some of my greatest meltdowns have happened after not getting dressed or putting on makeup for a week. I have acknowledged that, for myself, looking "nice" (aka getting dressed) helps keep me sane. Some of my friends never wear

[24] Serrallach, *Postnatal Depletion Cure*, 236.

makeup because that's not their thing, and I greatly respect them for that. I'm sure they have something else that they treat themselves to—maybe going for a run or using a good face lotion. Sometimes women use the term "self-care" as an excuse to indulge in their wants, but I am using self-care here to mean taking care of myself, so that I can take care of my family. Here are some self-care priorities I have developed for myself:

+ Shower and exercise.
+ Get dressed and put makeup on.
+ Read books before bed instead of staring at my phone.
+ Take some time each week for myself, to shop or run errands or just be by myself in a quiet place.
+ Use paper plates during busy times so there are fewer dishes to do.
+ If a friend offers to help, take her up on it.
+ Schedule nights out, or play dates in, with other moms to give me something to look forward to during the week.
+ Take naps. PBS Kids is educational! I can put the baby to bed, put on a show for the older kids, and nap right next to them. For me, a half-hour power nap can do wonders.

Your list will look different, but I encourage you to make a list. Don't neglect yourself to the detriment of your family.

Recognizing Triggers

One way I could tell I was struggling postpartum was that I was unable to accomplish seemingly small tasks. For example, mopping the floor was a chore that seemed too overwhelming. It required picking up everything off the floor, sweeping or vacuuming, and then pulling out my steam cleaner. If I didn't get every square inch clean, I felt it wouldn't have been a job well done. And instead of doing a "poor job," I just avoided doing it altogether.

Cleaning the floor should not be a monumental task, but when I was struggling with postnatal depletion, it was. When I finally came around to doing chores again, mopping became a little more regular, but I began to notice an interesting coincidence. There were some days that were particularly hard for my mental health. I didn't feel as if I could relax in my own home: there were too many things left undone, and I felt scatterbrained. These were also the days when I felt the sticky spots on the floor and crunched crumbs under my socks. But once I finally mopped the floor, I felt ten times better.

Now I know that, for me, a dirty floor is a mental-health trigger. The rest of the house can be a mess, but if the main floor is clean, I can have some peace. Every mother has her own trigger, but if you can find out what it is, you can make that task a priority.

7

Spiritual Life

The saints were those who sank themselves in their
work, and so sanctified both themselves and it.[25]

The "Unholy" Years

I spent a solid four years immersed in postpartum, pregnancy,
anxiety, and depression. There were some brighter moments
during those years, but they all had a dark cloud over them.
One of the worst parts of those years was my sense of spiritual
failure. I watched a lot of TV and did not do a lot of praying. I
did the minimum: Sunday Mass, twice-a-year Confession, and
some half-hearted prayers here and there. Every so often, I'd get
a little more serious, read a spiritual book, or read the daily Mass
readings. But compared with where I was before these pregnan-
cies, I felt disgusted at myself and unable to change.

Before I became a mother, I worked at a parish. From the time
I got serious about my faith in high school, I had always been
involved in ministry. I studied theology and catechetics in college

---

[25] Hubert van Zeller, *Holiness for Housewives (and Other Working
Women)* (Manchester, NH: Sophia Institute Press, 1997), 17.

and became a youth minister after I graduated. I went to daily Mass; I prayed in the adoration chapel. In short, my life revolved around being at church. It's even where I met my husband! And now, I was constantly at home with babies who seemed to be tearing me *away* from my spiritual life instead of making my life holier. I struggled with the guilt of not attending daily Mass, not having twenty minutes of quiet time a day, neglecting to say my morning offering, or going months without visiting the adoration chapel.

I knew motherhood was supposed to be good and holy, but it didn't feel that way to me. I wasn't doing all the external practices that used to make me feel like a good Catholic, so I kept my distance from God. Sure, there was Sunday Mass and my weekly mom's prayer group and the frantic "God help me!" shot toward heaven as the poop shot out toward the wall, or the midnight promise that I would say the Rosary more if only this child would go to sleep!

The devil wanted me to believe that this was a failure in prayer. He tried to make me think that God was disappointed in my efforts. In reality, God was trying to teach me something new in this season of life: that it's not all about me. I was, in fact, praying more often than I thought, only it didn't look the way it did when I was a youth minister. St. Thérèse wrote, "For me, prayer is a surge of the heart; it is a simple look turned toward heaven, it is a cry of recognition and of love, embracing both trial and joy."[26] I was looking toward heaven with a cry—that's for sure! And I was never more aware of my weaknesses and trials than during that time.

[26] CCC 2558, quoting St. Thérèse of Lisieux, *Manuscrits autobiographiques*, C 25r.

Weakness

What I couldn't see back then was that those longings to change, even if it felt as if nothing was happening, were indeed changing me over a period of years. In those days of glaring inadequacies, all I could bring to God were my deficiencies. What I didn't know was that those "nothings" were all that God wanted me to bring.

St. Faustina's spiritual director once told her, "Comport yourself before God like the widow in the Gospel; although the coin she dropped into the box was of little value, it counted far more before God than all the big offerings of others."[27]

The poor widow, the blind man, the beggar, the prostitute, the good thief: we were all coming to God totally inadequate with nothing grand to give. But that's precisely when God fills in those empty spaces with His grace and life. It's in our deficiencies that we give God room to work.

On the other hand, the rich man and the Pharisees: they thought they had it together because they followed the laws and had an impressive résumé of accomplishments. Only, Jesus couldn't care less about those accomplishments on their own; He wanted the gift of their whole being in love. He wanted the good and the bad, their successes *and* failures.

When we are filled with self, and think we've got this mothering thing down on our own, there is no room for God. When we are emptied of self, then God can fill us with His divine life. In the words of John the Baptist, "He must increase, but I must decrease" (John 3:30). It's in these times of postpartum motherhood that we experience this self-emptying so poignantly, yet

[27] Saint Maria Faustina Kowalska, *Divine Mercy in My Soul*, 3rd ed. (Stockbridge, MA: Congregation of Marians, 2003), 27.

too often we despair that things are not the way they used to be and conclude that we must be failing.

But what if that's just where God wants us to be? What if He wants it to seem as if we are failing at this mothering thing, just so we can realize how much we need Him, in the same way our babies rely on us to meet their needs?

One night, as I was journaling, I wrote that my faith is so weak. God spoke to me through Scripture and reminded me: "'My grace is sufficient for you, for my power is made perfect in weakness.' I will all the more gladly boast of my weaknesses, that the power of Christ may rest upon me" (2 Cor. 12:9).

When I am weak, then He is strong. A postpartum spirituality is the recognition that we are nothing without God. We must bring to God our nothingness and let Him fill the spaces with Himself; His divine life, His grace.

When I finally asked God if He wanted me to go to daily Mass with my four children under six, He didn't give me any indication that I should. He was asking me to be present to the needs of my small children, and in doing so, I would be showing Him love. It took me years to figure it out, but He was asking me to find His presence in the ordinary tasks of motherhood.

The Ordinary

In my seventh year of motherhood, with four children at home, my new spiritual director recommended that I read the book *The Reed of God* by Caryll Houselander. I had shared with this priest that I struggled to relate to Mary in my motherhood. She seemed aloof to me, too perfect to imitate. All my life I had wanted to love her as others around me did, but it didn't come easy. Then I read this book, and a whole new way of looking at Mary was opened to me.

Mary's life was actually very ordinary, much like mine. We don't know the details of her life, but we can imagine they were similar to ours—nursing in the middle of the night, teaching the baby Jesus to walk, talk, and obey Joseph. She was a homemaker, shopping in the village and preparing meals for her family. She supported Joseph in his work as a carpenter. Nazareth was a small, lowly town. Nothing good or fancy would come from there, others had said (see John 1:46). Caryll Houselander wrote:

> The one thing that He did ask of [Mary] was the gift of her humanity. She was to give Him her body and soul unconditionally, and ... she was to give Him her daily life.
>
> And outwardly it would not differ from the life she would have led if she had not been chosen to be the Bride of the Spirit and the Mother of God at all!
>
> She was not even asked to live it alone with this God who was her own Being and whose Being was to be hers. No, He asked for her ordinary life shared with Joseph....
>
> Yes, it certainly seemed that God wanted to give the world the impression that it is ordinary for Him to be born of a human creature.
>
> Well, that is a fact. God did mean it to be the ordinary thing, for it is His will that Christ shall be born in every human being's life and not, as a rule, through extraordinary things, but through the ordinary daily life and the human love that people give to one another.[28]

Even though, while caring for an infant, there are times when Christ seems far from you—you are hardly sleeping; you

---

[28] Caryll Houselander, *The Reed of God* (London: Sheed and Ward, 1978), 12.

are either shushing a crying baby or chasing a crawling toddler during Mass—and quiet time seems hard to come by, Christ is actually very near. Christ is as close to you as He was to Mary when she was caring for Him—changing His diapers and shushing His crying. To be like Christ is to grow in love, and other than the marital embrace, there is no human love like a mother's love for her child. She gives of herself over and over again, without asking anything in return. So that yes to God in caring for your children imitates Mary in her yes to God in caring for Jesus.

> Our Lady said yes for the human race. Each one of us must echo that yes for our own lives.
>
> We are all asked if we will surrender what we are, our humanity, our flesh and blood, to the Holy Spirit and allow Christ to fill the emptiness formed by the particular shape of our life.[29]

Finding God at Home

There are many people in the world who cultivate a curious state which they call "the spiritual life." They often complain that they have very little time to devote to the "spiritual life." The only time that they do not regard as wasted is the time they can devote to pious exercises: praying, reading, meditations, and visiting the church.

All the time spent in earning a living, cleaning the home, caring for the children, making and mending clothes, cooking, and all the other manifold duties

[29] Ibid., 13.

and responsibilities is regarded as wasted. Yet it is really
through ordinary human life and the things of every hour
of every day that union with God comes about.[30]

As my frame of mind shifted from praying in church to praying
at home, I had to figure out what that would look like. I now know
that if God wanted motherhood to be filled with holy hours and
church events, He wouldn't have created babies to be so needy.
But your baby needs you the way you need God, meaning all
the time! Then I came upon the book *Holiness for Housewives*,
written by Hubert van Zeller, a priest who was a spiritual director
to many housewives. His simple guidance helped me to see the
holiness in my everyday chores.

> The only thing that really matters in life is doing the will
> of God.... Your whole business is still to look for God in
> the midst of all this [housework, daily tasks, and so forth].
> You will not find Him anywhere else. If you leave your
> dishes, your housekeeping, your telephone calls, your
> children's everlasting questions, your ironing, and your
> invitations to take care of themselves while you go off and
> search for our Lord's presence in prayer, you will discover
> nothing but self....
>
> So it is idle for you to complain about the drawbacks
> to spirituality that you find in your particular vocation.
> There is nothing that you are up against that God has not
> given you the grace to surmount. You can, if you want,
> turn the monotony and the drudgery and the distraction
> into an expression of love.[31]

[30] Ibid., 5.
[31] Van Zeller, *Holiness for Housewives*, 13–14, 16.

In her diary, St. Faustina recounts her struggle, while on kitchen duty, to drain the pot of boiled potatoes. The pot was too heavy for her, and often the potatoes spilled out with the water. So she began to avoid the potatoes at all cost, and the sisters noticed. What they didn't notice was that St. Faustina was willing and wanted to drain the potatoes but lacked the strength. She prayed to God about her weakness, and He told her He would give her the strength starting tomorrow. The next day, St. Faustina volunteered to drain the potatoes and accomplished it with ease. When she lifted the lid, she discovered the pot was filled with roses, and she heard a voice within her say, *"I change such hard work of yours into bouquets of most beautiful flowers, and their perfume rises up to my throne."*[32]

Motherhood offers us the same opportunity: to turn our scrubbing toilets and changing diapers into bouquets of flowers. I was reminded of this once when I was steam cleaning the floors and Timothy, a five-year-old at the time, saw the steam rising off the mop head. He told me that if I put prayers on the steam, they would rise to heaven like incense. How wonderful a thought — my prayers rising to heaven on steam while I clean the floor!

"Your whole purpose, then, is to work out a way of praying that directs every effort towards God — and to work out a way of directing effort so that everything becomes a prayer."[33]

And even though the quiet times seem few and far between, I have surprisingly discovered over the years that there is a lot of time to be contemplative in raising children, as my thoughts rise to heaven while I do my ordinary, everyday chores.

[32] Saint Faustina Kowalska, *Divine Mercy*, no. 33.
[33] Van Zeller, *Holiness for Housewives*, 26.

Control

The postpartum season of spiritual growth is deeply interior and has less to do with our external efforts. If anything, this season teaches us to give up control. We are not in control of our children's sleeping habits or appetites or the timing of their diaper changes. What I felt the Holy Spirit telling me after Zoe's birth was "Stop trying to control everything!" But we love control: to control our fertility and to stay on schedule for our careers and retirement. We want three easy steps to sleep training, potty-training in a day, and if we could just instill virtues in our kids by the time they are four years old, that would be great. Then we can be finished with our part, send them to school, and call it good.

Unfortunately, there is no secret to easy, successful parenting no matter what the experts say. It's a slow trial and error. (I quickly decided to throw out all my books by "experts" shortly after Timothy was born.) Sure, there may be tips to help your baby sleep, but there is no guarantee. And your baby may be a good eater until he starts teething and then all bets are off. Meanwhile, virtues need to be taught over and over again until adulthood! It's about surrendering to the schedule and needs of your children instead of your own.

The postpartum stage doesn't need to be a time to double down on your prayer schedule, but a chance to allow your baby to reveal to you the love of the Father. The unconditional love I have for my children is just a glimpse of the merciful love the Father has for me. No matter how frustrated I am with a child or how mad I am that the baby is not sleeping, when my children look at me and smile, I am filled with love for them. No matter how gross a child's diaper just was, I am happy to hold and cuddle him or her (once the diaper is changed). There's nothing I won't do for my babies! In the same way, no matter what I've done or said, or how bad I think I've failed, God wants me to turn to Him so He can forgive me and show me His love.

I think this is the key to postpartum spirituality: to allow the Lord to lead you through your child's needs. It's not laziness or giving up when you are intentionally surrendering to the work of the Spirit. A wise priest once said, "When you get up at night to take care of your baby, you are doing for your baby what God does for us. Being faithful to the duties of your state is more pleasing to God than hours of adoration." The year after having a baby is a demanding season of life, but we can change and grow right along with our babies if we are open to the Spirit and allow the Lord to work through our mothering.

In *On the Other Side of Fear*, Hallie Lord writes:

> What I've slowly come to understand is that these cold, dark seasons are not useless. They don't point to a failure on my part to be holy. If anything, they make me more honest. They strip me of platitudes and false humility and bring me to my knees before God, pummeling the dirt with my fists and settling the dust with my tears. They strip me of pride and, left completely spent and with nowhere else to turn, lift my lined face toward my Maker.
>
> These seasons are not prayer-schedule friendly, but they are every bit as essential to spiritual growth as the seasons that allow me to meditate deeply for long periods of time. These are the seasons that teach me to let go and surrender. And if the years since my conversion have taught me anything, it is that spiritual growth is synonymous with spiritual surrender.[34]

---

[34] Hallie Lord, *On the Other Side of Fear: How I Found Peace* (Huntington, IN: Our Sunday Visitor, 2016), 98–99.

I now see that, initially, I made prayer all about me and my efforts to get to God. My pride got in the way of the surrender required for real conversion. The underlying desire was good (i.e., to get to God), but what God showed me was that my greatest efforts alone are still puny. Prayer is all about making ourselves available for God to come to us, and the postpartum years taught me how to surrender. I can surrender and open myself up to Him while doing dishes or laundry or while reading a story to my kids. I can sweep the floor for love of Jesus just as St. Thérèse did.

You can meet God in the depth of your heart, no matter what you are doing, and it's the continual union with God throughout the day that helps you to grow in holiness. If you can quiet your soul and learn to recognize God's voice through meditating on the Scriptures, you'll be surprised at how much He is saying to you.

In fact, in the years of early motherhood, I heard God's voice most often in the shower. At the end of the day, all alone with the sound of the water acting as white noise to my distracted thoughts, I would hear Him whisper into my heart.

Daily Sacrifices

During my ups and downs of prayer, I did not fail the basic precepts of the Church. We went to Mass every Sunday (even if we had to go separately on occasion to leave the kids at home) and on holy days of obligation. I was there with my two small coins (and small babies). Ever since I had my first child, though, I've had trouble paying attention at Mass because someone always needs something. And although I initially felt guilty about being distracted, I now know that my gift is the offering of myself, however closely I am able to pay attention.

What I began to realize on retreat with Fr. Riley is that through my Baptism, I was also baptized into the royal priesthood. The common priesthood (as opposed to the ministerial priesthood) is what all Catholics are baptized into, meaning that we share in Christ's death and Resurrection with every sacrifice we make, joining our offerings in the sacrifice of the Eucharist. This means that every Sunday, I bring the sacrifices of that past week and lay them at the altar, whether I am able to pay attention fully to the readings or not. Just as Christ's sacrifice on the Cross was redemptive, my sufferings, united to His, have redemptive value, too.

Daily sacrifices joined to Christ's one sacrifice give new meaning to every difficulty I face: a teething baby who won't nap, cleaning up vomit, pen on the couch, night feedings, children's tantrums while I'm trying to make dinner. When I pay attention, I realize that taking care of babies and small children means that I have plenty to offer up throughout the day. I can offer up sacrifices and sufferings for my family, for the intentions of a friend, for the intentions of the Church, for the conversion of sinners, for the souls in purgatory, or for anyone who needs prayer.

Confession

For a few years, I did the basic twice-a-year Confession during Lent and Advent. It seemed so hard to get away from the babies to go stand in line for Confession, or 3:00 p.m. on a Saturday would come and go without my even thinking about it. And yet, I could find time to get away to have a drink with a friend or go shopping by myself. I have to admit: it was my priorities.

Then Fr. Riley put it this way: Would you bathe only twice a year? You would stink! How much more do our souls need to bathe in the grace of the sacrament of Reconciliation! If I really felt that way about having a clean soul, I would make time for it or put it on my calendar so I wouldn't forget! What reasons should I have for not availing myself of the mercy of God? I hate waiting in line? I have a baby?! When I realized I was using my baby as my excuse for not going to Confession, I knew this had to change. I now have a goal to make it every two or three months. Even with a baby, I think this is attainable!

Speaking of grace and being disposed to receive it, a sacramental that I put off for way too long was getting our house blessed. Our house was always under construction, so I thought we'd have it done "when this project is done" or "when this priest is available." I wanted it to include a nice dinner and be a big to-do, so I kept putting it off. We lived in our house for four years before getting it blessed. As I look back at all my mental and spiritual struggles during this time, I wish I had asked for God's blessing on our house much sooner. The devil is prowling, looking for someone to devour. He certainly got to devour a lot of my thoughts, and I needed as much protection as possible!

Prayer

In addition to the sacraments, I found that there were some prayers that could easily be fit into my day as a mother, and that the small effort to pray them did help me raise my mind to God. I don't say all these prayers every day, but I draw from this list to find ways to open my heart to God in and through my motherhood.

Morning offering

For a while, I had a printed morning offering placed in my cabinet above the coffee maker. Since drinking coffee was the one thing I did regularly each morning without fail, I figured that having my morning offering right there would help me pray it without fail as well. Well, it failed.

Then I printed a prettier (but harder to read) version of the morning offering and placed it behind my kitchen sink, next to the plant I never watered. Finally, I put it on my dresser, where I straighten my hair and put on makeup each morning. Yet I still didn't stop and say the whole dang prayer! It made me feel so guilty that the whole morning had gone by, and I hadn't stopped to read the offering, even though I still directed my thoughts to God each morning and throughout my day.

Then a priest told me that it's okay to make up our own morning offering. In fact, it's a really good thing to be able to pray in our own words! So now I say, either as I open my eyes in bed or walk down the hall to the coffee machine, "God, I give this day to You." And after I've had my coffee, I can add to that prayer any other prayers (written or in my own words).

There is certainly a place for recited communal prayer, such as the Rosary, the Mass, and the Liturgy of the Hours. But what Catholics often seem to lack is the heart of prayer, the union of our hearts to God's. Composing prayers from the heart in our own words is also essential to a deep spiritual life, and postpartum is a great season of life to practice those spontaneous prayers, those cries of the heart, such as, "God, I need you! I am nothing without you."

Decades of the Rosary

A decade of the Rosary takes only a couple of minutes. And because I have ten fingers, it's possible to pray a decade anytime and anywhere if I give it some thought. When I was a new mother, I figured that nursing would be a good time to pray the Rosary. Well, that didn't work out very well. My mind wanders, and I space out during nursing. I had to let go of the expectation that that would be a good time to pray. But if I can pray a decade a day for five days, then I have prayed a Rosary! And what better way to embrace motherhood than by meditating on the motherhood of Mary and entrusting our lives to her care.

"Harvard-trained cardiologist and professor Herbert Benson coined the term 'relaxation response' after discovering that you can calm yourself when you consciously let go of all thoughts and actively engage in a repetitive activity. A state of relaxation is when your nervous system is reset to a neutral position."[35] Guess what is a calm and repetitive activity? Praying the Rosary! So is washing dishes, showering, folding clothes, and a lot of other household tasks.

Adoration

During the 2018 "summer of scandal," I became really anxious reading news article after news article about abuse among the clergy. One night, I went to a Q and A on the abuse crisis, hosted by some priests and diocesan workers. After talking about the abuse for almost an hour, one of the priests brought out the Blessed Sacrament. The difference I felt in my soul was like night and day—from anxiety to peace. I knew the problems weren't solved, but I also felt palpably that Jesus is King and He reigns. When He says, "Come to me and I will give you rest," He means it. There have been several times since when I have entered into the adoration chapel after a noisy day, and that contrasting peace again was there. I can't recommend the meditation that yoga offers, but I can wholeheartedly endorse the peace that comes from Christ Himself.

[35] Serrallach, *Postnatal Depletion Cure*, 25.

The Sacred Heart

I love the Sacred Heart and have had a strong devotion to it ever since high school. As one who feels things deeply, the image is a reminder that Christ feels things deeply, too. The flames on top, the drops of blood, and the thorns surrounding the Heart are all such vivid images of Christ's passionate love for us. When I feel lonely or sad, I imagine myself crawling into the slit in the side of His Heart and resting inside. I join with St. Faustina in saying, "Oh, how great is the fire of purest love which burns in Your Most Sacred Heart! Happy the soul that has come to understand the love of the Heart of Jesus!"[36]

Divine Mercy

I also have in my house an image of Divine Mercy, with the words, "Jesus, I trust in You" underneath. It's near my kitchen, so I try to glance at the picture during the day to remind me of Jesus' love for me. The pale ray represents the water that makes souls righteous, and the red ray stands for Jesus' Blood, which is the life of souls. As I see the rays pouring out from Jesus' Heart and His hands open wide, it looks as if Jesus is giving His grace and mercy directly to me, and so He is. It's nothing I deserve but everything I need. When I am tempted by anxious thoughts, I often cry out, "Jesus, I trust in You!"

The Jesus Prayer

The Jesus Prayer is simple: "Jesus Christ, Son of God, have mercy on me, a sinner." You are supposed to say it slowly and quietly and pause to take a deep breath after every phrase. Inhaling and exhaling while praying this prayer calms the mind until it rests on Jesus.

[36] Saint Faustina Kowalska, *Divine Mercy*, no. 141.

[The Jesus Prayer] combines the Christological hymn of Philippians 2:6–11 with the cry of the publican and the blind men begging for light (cf. Mark 10:46–52; Luke 18:13). By it the heart is opened to human wretchedness and the Savior's mercy.

The invocation of the holy name of Jesus is the simplest way of praying always. When the holy name is repeated often by a humbly attentive heart, the prayer is not lost by heaping up empty phrases (cf. Matt. 6:7), but holds fast to the word and "brings forth fruit with patience" (Luke 8:15). This prayer is possible "at all times" because it is not one occupation among others but the only occupation: that of loving God, which animates and transfigures every action in Christ Jesus. (CCC 2667–2668)

If you can't seem to pray any other prayer during the day, say the name of Jesus.

Daily Mass readings

The one thing I've tried to be consistent with is reading the daily readings for Mass along with the rest of the universal Church. Scripture is the living Word of God, and what better way to be attentive to God than to hear His words directly? My husband and I often read them together while drinking coffee before he goes to work, but sometimes I read them on my own later in the day. I also love the "Blessed Is She" reflections, e-mailed daily, as a great way of breaking open the daily Scriptures with other Catholic women.

Examen

When all else fails and the day is almost at an end, you still have the moments before falling asleep to raise your thoughts to God as you reflect on your day. The Examen is a habit of prayer that St. Ignatius of Loyola shared with his followers, and one that anyone can practice in five steps:[37]

1. Invite the Holy Spirit into your thoughts as you become aware of God's presence. Ask God for clarity and understanding.
2. Review the day with gratitude. Focus on the people you interacted with, the work you did, and the small things you experienced, with gratefulness for all God's gifts.
3. Pay attention to your thoughts and emotions of the day. Bring those feelings to God, and ask Him what you can learn from them.
4. Ask forgiveness for your sins and shortcomings.
5. Look toward tomorrow. Seek God's guidance for the tasks and decisions ahead. End with the Our Father.

[37] "How Can I Pray?" IgnatianSpirituality.com, https://www.ignatianspirituality.com/ignatian-prayer/the-examen/how-can-i-pray.

8

Community and Identity

I was sitting at my dining room table in my pajamas, my dirty hair up in a bun (and not a fashionable "messy bun"), and staring at my sister-in-law across the table through my puffy, sleep-deprived eyes. She had a two-year-old and a three-month-old, and I had only a two-month-old. She sat there with her makeup perfectly applied, hair curled by a curling iron, and a cute, stylish outfit on that didn't scream "post-maternity clothes." I couldn't understand how I hardly had time to take a shower and she had double the kids I did, yet she still made it out of the house looking like a million bucks. In fact, I couldn't even make it out of the house: she came to me.

After four kids, I have finally come to accept that I don't bounce back after having a baby. My saggy belly two years later is proof of that. It takes me a few months to feel even remotely normal again. For me, the first big milestone is at two months, when I can formulate a coherent sentence. The next is at four months, when I can walk out of the house with makeup and decent clothes on. And really, it isn't until nine months postpartum that I welcome my husband's embrace and feel ready to engage with the outside world.

Other mothers ask me which of my four births was the most difficult transition. Zero to one? One to two? Typically, my answer is that each transition is hard! They all have their difficult moments, such as the firsts with your first or running out of arms with your third.

This past summer, we were flying to Oregon for vacation, and we met a young family on the underground train to our terminal. The mother had a two-year-old and an infant and saw that I was sitting with Luke and Zoe. The mother commented on my two kids, and I replied, "Oh, we actually have four," and as others got off the train, my husband moved over next to us with the older two. You could see her eyes go wide as she shared with me, "I always thought I wanted three kids, but now I'm not so sure . . ." she trailed off. I assured her that she was in the thick of it: having a toddler and an infant is the most exhausting phase with kids. As she watched my kids giggle with each other and talk excitedly about the plane ride, I hope she was able to see how lovely siblings can be in a few years, even if it's hard at the moment. They don't stay babies forever.

Having mom friends gives us perspective. I can look at a friend whose kids are older than mine and see how fast our kids really do grow and change in such a short time. I can complain about teething or naps, and another mom can remind me of how quickly a baby's sleep schedule changes.

We need real, authentic relationships with other moms in order to survive this wild, chaotic ride called motherhood, especially during the postpartum time. Social media gets blamed for a lot of our unrealistic expectations, yet some of this blame is accurate. I do not have accounts on Instagram or Pinterest, because I know myself, and I can't handle comparing myself with those picture-perfect snapshots of life. It's when I go over to my friends' houses, with crumbs on the floor and their kids' hair as nappy as my own kids' hair, that I feel as if I've come to the right place. We can't have it all together all the time, and we shouldn't be expected to.

Finding Community

After Timothy was born, I felt terribly alone. Many of my good friends at the time were still single and working during the day when I was at home with the baby. I found a moms' group forty minutes away that I would drive to every other week, but everyone there was already friends, and I didn't find a welcoming community.

After Lily was born and I was in my darkest hour of nursing and thrush and depression, I e-mailed the group, asking for prayers and sharing some of what was going on. Almost immediately meals came pouring in, and I was so grateful for the support. Although I didn't know these women well, they knew motherhood well and could offer a hand when I needed it most. That year, the group disbanded.

I knew from that glimpse of community that I needed a moms' group, but I didn't know of any that were closer to home. So I gathered together a friend or two and called a few of the nearby parishes to see if they would host a moms' group. Most parishes liked the idea but didn't have the facilities or the resources to accommodate us. But one parish already had a nursery and was very open to the idea, as they had a dwindling women's Rosary group that had been meeting there for years and using their nursery. The other leader and I combined to form the Rosary Moms' Group, which was marked by praying the Rosary together, inviting speakers, having brunches, and doing book studies. The word spread, the group grew, and it was a huge blessing that once a week I would drop my kids off in the nursery and share in prayer and fellowship with other moms.

Deep Friendship

When Nathan and I started talking about buying a house, we were looking all over the Denver metro area. The one thing I always considered, though, was how far away a potential home was from my moms' group. It had been my lifeline for two years, and I couldn't imagine surviving without it.

After we moved to the other side of town, I continued to drive to the group for a while. Not only was I always late, but I found that I only saw these women during moms' group time. As the group had changed, I no longer had deep friendships with any of the members in which we shared our hearts and had phone conversations and got our kids together for playdates.

There were so many difficult times in the transition of moving and having Luke that I just needed someone to talk to. I called my mom a lot, but there are some things I'd just rather not talk about with her. I felt so alone and terribly stuck. I had a moment in my kitchen, sobbing, where I begged God to send me a friend. *Just one friend, Lord, for me to talk to in these difficult moments.* For months I prayed this prayer, and after about a year, it was finally answered. And it was answered in not one friend, but two! God had heard my prayer, but He had to wait to answer it until these women moved to town. And He can never be outdone in generosity!

I like to joke that making new friends as a mom is like dating all over again. You do your hair, dress in your nicest clothes, and pull out your best parenting tricks to make a good impression.

You exchange numbers and start texting. Then comes the big day when you invite this friend over for coffee or a playdate. You clean furiously before she comes over. After she leaves, you agonize over every detail and wonder if there will ever be a follow-up coffee.

Sometimes the two of you click, and the friendship works out. Sometimes you realize that although you both have the best intentions, your lives or personalities are just too different. That's okay too. But the only way to make friends is to put yourself out there, join a group at church (or start one!), or even just walk over to someone at the park and introduce yourself. For introverts like me, it can take quite a bit of energy and effort in the beginning, but the community that comes from it is definitely worth it in the end.

As friends move away or drift apart, I find I'm never done being open to new friendships. Something that became important to Nathan and me while remodeling our house was our family mission to be welcoming and to build community. We try to have a family over for dinner at least once a month, in order to make connections and encourage relationships among spouses and children.

Comparison

C. S. Lewis wrote in his book *Mere Christianity*, "How gloriously different are the saints."[38] I love to read the lives of the saints, and it's true that no two are alike. Coming from different continents and speaking different languages, the Communion of Saints

[38] C. S. Lewis, *Mere Christianity* (New York: Macmillan, 1960), 190.

comprises kings and queens, peasants and servants, priests and nuns of all different religious orders, married people and children. Some were martyred, others died of sickness, and the list goes on.

In my experience, the same is true for women: how gloriously different are all the mothers! The truth is, there is more than one right way to do things, just as there is more than one right path to holiness: hospital birth versus home birth; breastfeeding versus bottle feeding; swaddles versus swings; working versus staying at home. One time, the Internet went crazy over how often children should have a bath. Everything depends on your personality, your child's temperament, and your unique circumstances.

C. S. Lewis's premise is that when we give ourselves entirely over to Christ, He fills us with His personality, of which there is no end to the variation. He compares the way the Author creates each one of us unique to the way an author invents characters in a novel: "There is so much of Him that millions and millions of 'little Christs,' all different, will still be too few to express Him fully."[39]

Only, we have to give up ourselves to find our true selves in Christ. "It is no good trying to 'be myself' without Him," writes C. S. Lewis. If we are too focused on who we are trying to become, we will fall flat. "The same principle holds, you know, for everyday matters. Even in social life, you will never make a good impression on other people until you stop thinking about what sort of impression you are making."[40]

I've come to understand that the underlying reason we mothers compare ourselves with one another and put each other down is because we are insecure in our mothering and want to justify

[39] Ibid., 189.
[40] Ibid., 190.

our own choices, but this only hurts the community of women all struggling to do the right thing. It damages the Body of Christ because we are not meant to be one size fits all, but rather, unique expressions of the Infinite God. It is the devil who wants us divided.

I think back to the story of Cain and Abel. Cain compared his gift with that of his brother and became resentful and jealous. Yet we keep repeating the same sin, even though God has reminded us over and over again that He loves each of us infinitely, regardless of the size of our offering.

Moreover, God created us unique so that we would share our gifts with each other. Fr. Riley said: "It's called interdependency: God gives us different gifts because He wants us to work together. Don't be tempted to envy what another mother has. Whatever gift God has given you, use it to the best of your ability."

I currently stay at home and homeschool. But I have had several part-time jobs over the years. My sister is a full-time teacher with five kids. I know stay-at-home moms who send their kids to school, and I know moms who work as doctors or nurses or lawyers and hire nannies. I also know moms who work hard just to make ends meet. I rejoice for each mother's commitment to her children, regardless of her family's choices. Often, the ones who work struggle to balance their family lives, and sometimes the ones who don't work struggle to balance their finances or their personal lives. It doesn't mean that any of these are bad choices; it just means that these moms are different from their neighbors. The most important choices involve seeking God's will, loving your family to the best of your ability, and striving to use the unique gifts God has given you to build up His kingdom here on earth, whether it's with ten people or ten hundred.

Baby and Beyond

Identity

I have had many conversations with friends in recent years about finding ourselves after having kids. It's so easy to lose our identity because we become absorbed in our kids' needs and schedules. But it's not selfish to develop your own skills and talents. In fact, if you do, you are likely to inspire your kids to follow their own dreams and use the gifts that God has given them.

After doing my stint as the hospitality coordinator at our parish, I realized that hospitality to the masses was not my gift. As an introvert who prefers small-group settings, the experience drained me. After I quit, I asked God what my gifts were, and I heard very clearly that they were writing and teaching. Shortly afterward, I got a part-time job doing just that—teaching for CatholicMarriagePrep.com as an online instructor and writing for its blog. That work filled me and gave me an outlet. Two years later, our family was bigger, my husband's business was picking up, and we were getting serious about homeschooling, so I discerned that my gift of teaching would be best used right then for my children. And then God placed the vision of this book on my heart, and I began to write as well.

Having Hobbies

At a baby shower before Timothy was born, I was given a gift certificate to a bookstore. Timothy was two months old when I strolled him up to the store. A book on the clearance rack just outside the front door caught my eye: *The Cake Mix Doctor*. As I flipped through the pages, I saw fancy and delicious cakes all made easy by beginning with a cake mix. My mom baked a lot when I was growing up, and I have fond memories of decorating cakes and cookies with her. I was spending so much time home alone while Timothy was napping that I needed a hobby, so I took up baking. I made my way through parts of the cake book for birthdays, guests, and even just because. This hobby didn't do anything to help me lose the baby weight, but it did build confidence in my cooking skills so I could be a better host for friends and family. It also became a tradition to let the kids pick out the cakes they'd like me to make for their birthdays.

I used to be envious of my husband's hobbies, such as golf, snowboarding, fishing, and woodworking. They were all so concrete, while I didn't feel I had any one hobby that was my thing. Talking one morning over omelets, a friend of mine shared the same struggle. She had recently read Jennifer Fulwiler's book *One Beautiful Dream* and was trying to figure out her "blue flame." My friend and I had both been in ministry during our college years, and youth ministers after college, and being in ministry was when we really came alive. Now, in our years of young motherhood, God was asking us to be home with our children, and we were looking for ways to find our flame, or passion, which would fill us up and allow us to come back to our family refreshed.

As we talked, she realized that perhaps she didn't have just one passion, but that she needed a chunk of time each month to do one of the many things she loves: decorating, thrift-store shopping, or meeting up with friends for a deep heart-to-heart. Community is important to her, and she still shares her love of Christ in her women's group and in their family group. Currently, she is beginning a social media initiative called The Vows Project to encourage and strengthen marriages, combining her passion for the faith with her life as a mother and wife.

I have found a similar pattern in my life: meeting up with friends and sharing our hearts over a glass of wine or a cup of espresso, exploring new sights around Colorado with my family, and reading good books are all "hobbies" that make me come alive. I still love to bake and cook, but as my family grows in size and the dishes grow in piles, it's not always the fun outlet that it used to be. It's now a necessity to feed my family, and an act of love to make something delicious that my husband will enjoy.

Finally, I have discovered that as my children get older, I am able to share my hobbies with them. I find joy in teaching my kids and learning right along with them. They bake alongside me in the kitchen, and we have begun to explore new trails in the Colorado Rockies together.

Hidden Life

During the six years that I birthed four children, I went through a kind of identity crisis. When I thought back to my life before kids, I felt that I used to be so adventurous and full of life. Then, when I looked at my life with kids, I felt so stuck—as in: I'm just changing diapers, feeding people, washing dishes, and doing laundry on repeat. Is this what I have become? Is this what the rest of my life is doomed to look like?

And yet, when I look more closely at my life and my identity, I see that although a lot has changed, the core of me is still the same. While in prayer, I thought about the tiny mustard seed. Small and insignificant, it lies dormant in the ground. But while it is hidden there, a new life begins. Eventually the seed no longer looks like a seed but grows into a mighty tree.

My life does look different than before I had kids, but as I went through that identity crisis, I realized that I'm growing into a tree. Throughout the hidden postpartum time, my life has been sprouting into a flourishing motherhood. I like to compare my life to the thirty years Jesus spent living a hidden life, and how the ordinary tasks of life prepared Him for His mission.

I also consider the hidden years of postpartum motherhood similar to the desert, stripping me of my false comforts and idols and showing me the necessity of faith in Jesus Christ. All the great prophets, such as Moses, Elijah, John the Baptist, and even Jesus Himself, spent time in the desert before beginning their ministries.

As Bishop Robert Barron put it in one of his daily reflections:

What does the desert symbolize? Confrontation with one's own sin; seeing one's dark side; a deep realization of one's dependency upon God; an ordering of the priorities of one's life; a simplification, a getting back to basics. It means any and all of these things. But the bottom line is that they are compelled to wait, during a time and in a place where very little life seems to be on offer. But it is precisely in such deserts that the flowers bloom.[41]

Postpartum motherhood requires getting back to basics and ordering priorities. I may not be as adventurous as I was before having children, but I am more courageous in other ways and a lot less selfish than I used to be. I am the most influential person in my children's lives, not only by meeting their basic needs but also by forming their characters and introducing them to God. I also know God's love in a deeper way than I used to. I value community and strive to build authentic relationships. I'm more grateful for the little blessings in life than I was before.

[41] *Daily Gospel Reflections from Bishop Barron*, Word on Fire Catholic Ministries, January 2, 2019.

Baby and Beyond

And far from my life being over now that I have kids (as my melancholic nature tends to think), it's really just beginning. I think about how Mother Teresa was over forty when she founded the Missionaries of Charity, and St. John Paul II became pope when he was fifty-eight! God often works in us slowly, over time, just as the mighty oak in my neighbor's yard took sixty years to reach its current size. It takes time to flourish fully.

My children are preparing me for something great, whether here on earth or in heaven. When I stop to look, I see how these tiny human beings increase my capacity to love, teach me virtue, and make my world a better place with their enthusiasm and wonder. I tend easily to focus on the negative—the whining, crying, tantrums, and so much laundry! But now I work hard to focus more on the positive. The daily duties of hidden motherhood are slowly revealing my identity and my mission, so I can bloom and share my gifts with the world.

Meeting Each Other's Needs

When Zoe was six months old, I went out to eat with a friend for my birthday. Sitting in her car with bellies full of cheesecake, we lingered before heading into the clothing store to do some shopping. Well, to be more accurate, we never made it into the store because the tears started flowing as I shared with her the most intimate secret that I felt I had ever shared: sex was painful. All my feelings of being inadequate and alone came to the surface. How many times have I sobbed in my kitchen alone during naptime, feeling like the only wife in the world who struggled in the bedroom.

Much to my surprise, she said she had the same struggles in her marriage. She and her husband talk about it and work on it, but it's a cross. That conversation didn't solve my marital intimacy problems, but it did give me support and an outlet. Bolstered with courage from that conversation, I finally made an appointment with my doctor to get help.

Besides nutrient depletion and not taking time to rest and recover after delivery, not having a good sense of community is one of the other main reasons I believe women struggle so much after having a baby. We feel we are alone, as if we are the only ones struggling, and we have no one to share our deepest thoughts with. Dr. Serrallach shared in his book that as he researched other cultures, many had longstanding traditions in which family members came and took care of the cooking and the cleaning for the first month so that a mother who had just had a baby could focus on resting and nursing. In that time, a lot of wisdom can be passed on from one family member to the next.

One day, when I was praying the mystery of the Visitation (a decade here and there, right?), it struck me that even Mary, who had already said yes to being the Mother of God, still had to learn how to take care of a baby, and thus came to Elizabeth. Elizabeth also needed someone to help take care of her and her baby, and so the experience was mutual. We should be teaching each other the ropes of motherhood, while recognizing the beauty and creativity of our own personal journeys. Motherhood is not something that should be done alone.

Nowadays, we usually say no when someone asks to help us. We are embarrassed to admit we need help! And if you are like me, you don't usually think to offer help to someone else, either. One day after Zoe was born, my friend Heather called me up and said she was taking her kids to the park and offered to take mine as well so they could get some fresh air while I took a nap. By my fourth child, I knew better than to refuse help of this magnitude. She came over and took them, and it was grand. I wouldn't have asked her to take my kids to the park, but I was happy to take her up on it when she offered.

One of the greatest ways my community has helped me after I had a baby is with meals. At our moms' group, someone was in charge of organizing a meal train after a mother had a baby. Friends can go online and sign up for a day to bring a meal. With my last two children, I had meals made for us almost every other day for a month. Not only that, but most of the time there were leftovers for this starving, nursing mama to have for lunch the next day (or in the middle of the night). To know that other mothers were supporting me by dropping off meals lifted a huge burden; not only did I not have to shop or cook so much, but I knew I wasn't in this alone. There is a sense of camaraderie present through helping one another in that time of need.

Admitting We Can't Do It All

Although motherhood is an amazingly rich and satisfying experience like no other, it will always send you off on a twisting, turning road where you'll encounter bumps that you can't foresee. This is due to the physical changes that took place in your brain when you were pregnant, an overnight change in your relationship with your partner, social expectations that you can "do it all," hyper-vigilance in worrying about infant caretaking, sleep deprivation, hormonal shifts, physical depletion, and social isolation.[42]

Here in America, we mothers take pride in doing it all ourselves. My husband takes no time off after a baby comes. He is

[42] Serrallach, *Postnatal Depletion Cure*, 222.

self-employed, so if he doesn't work, we don't get paid. In the rare event that a friend offers to help us out, it's easy to decline. We think that asking for help is admitting weakness.

We also tend to think that a nanny is only for the rich (and how I wish I could afford one!). I have had a few friends tell me after their third or fourth babies that they hired a house cleaner every other week. They felt guilty spending money on that luxury, as if they were a failure for not being able to clean their own houses. I told them that if they have the money and the need, do it and don't feel guilty about it! There is nothing wrong with admitting we can't do it all and hiring help when we can afford it (which gives someone else work, too). For example, St. Zélie Martin (St. Thérèse of Lisieux's mom) hired a nanny while running her own lace-making business! We cannot do it all by ourselves.

Advice

Mothers get an overwhelming amount of unsolicited advice when they have a baby: how to get the baby to sleep, how often the baby should eat, when the baby should be lifting his head and crawling, and so forth. I'm not one who likes being told what to do. Amid my generally melancholic nature is a very definitive choleric streak. When most people give me advice, I nod, say thanks, and do the exact opposite of what they recommend. Still, I have heard three key pieces of wisdom over the years that were worthwhile:

1. *Admit when you are in survival mode.* This curbs the "feeling like a failure" guilt that often plagues the postpartum mom. I had one older homeschooling mom tell me that a few years back her family had a difficult year of big crises. The kids pretty much

watched TV all year long. When they got out of crisis mode, they resumed schooling and are now fine, not uneducated or addicted to the TV. That's more of an extreme example, but the reality is that when you have a baby, you are in survival mode. Lower your expectations. Then, after a year or so, when life is more manageable, declare yourself out of survival mode and make some intentional decisions to begin good habits, one at a time.

2. *Parenting turns a corner when your oldest turns five(ish)*. It's not a magical transformation on the morning of your child's fifth birthday, but I have noticed that children become a little bit more reasonable sometime after that birthday. If you have a baby, or two children under the age of three, you may see a big family with well-dressed children who behave at Mass and arrive on time. I'm telling you, do not compare yourself with them! As the older ones become, well, older, they will be more independent and helpful. It changes the dynamic. If that is not you, don't worry: your children will grow up. Right now, just make sure your toddler has two shoes on, even if the shoes don't match.

3. *Remember that babies' habits are only temporary*. A baby changes a lot in the first year, and so do his or her sleeping and eating schedules. Whatever habits a baby currently has (good or bad) will probably change in a few weeks. This summer, I had a friend over who had a five-year-old, a three-year-old, and an eleven-month-old with her. The older two went off to play with my kids, while the baby just crawled around on the floor under the table. My friend was venting about her baby's catnaps. "He's up before six and takes only two forty-five-minute catnaps. I know he's tired, but he just won't sleep any longer! I don't ever remember my older girls napping like this."

I asked her how long it had been going on. "A couple of days" was her reply.

"Has he been learning any new skills?" I asked.

"Yes, he's been pulling himself up to standing and walking along the furniture," she said.

"I remember complaining of Zoe's catnaps a year ago at this exact same time. I think it must be too exciting to stand, so they don't sleep as much. Give it a little more time, two weeks at most, and I'll bet he'll start sleeping better."

Communal Prayer

When I was attending the Rosary moms' group, I would drop my kids off in the nursery and pray the Rosary with a bunch of other moms once a week. I rarely prayed the Rosary on my own at this point, but gathering together with a bunch of other young moms ensured that I would do it weekly, encouraged by other women.

Now I go to an evening prayer group with other moms. We begin in the chapel with adoration and reflection on the upcoming Sunday's readings, and then we share about what God is doing in our hearts and what He is saying to us through those readings. Sometimes we pray over each other. Although I might not get to adoration very often on my own, I know I will go to adoration on those nights, praying alongside other women who have the same desire for holiness.

I am grateful to these groups of women for helping me to establish some habits of prayer. Time spent with the Blessed Sacrament in adoration or at Mass gives me the strength to remain united with Christ during my daily tasks for the rest of the week. Time spent praying the Rosary with other women helped me to invite the Blessed Mother to assist me in my mothering, surrounded by all these other mothers. But other than the encouragement to grow spiritually, the greatest gift from these communities of women has been learning to be vulnerable.

Vulnerability

The key to building authentic community is the ability to be vulnerable. Writing this book has been a very personal experience, one that wouldn't have been possible until I learned to be vulnerable and share my deepest thoughts and feelings with other mothers. "The village" doesn't magically appear after you have a baby; that is, people don't anticipate your needs and take care of you for months. Older cultures used to have those customs in place, but not today in America. Postpartum motherhood, especially if you've just had your first or second baby, can be one of the most lonely experiences in your life. I know; I've been there.

And yet that doesn't mean the village can't be built; it just means we have to be intentional about it. It takes one person to lay down her guard and open up first. It takes another person to receive that vulnerability and lay down her guard in return. From there, you can share on a deeply personal level about your fears and failures, you can ask for help or for prayers, and you can meet the physical needs of other mothers: a meal, babysitting, a pedicure, or a shoulder to cry on. And so the village is built, and authentic community begins to happen.

If we pretend that we've got it together and don't let anyone else see us for who we truly are — strengths and weaknesses — then we risk not being truly known or loved. The sad reality is that we can hide behind a smile at the park or on social media, and others might never know otherwise, unless we tell them. As I have begun to share the struggles I faced during my postpartum years, I've had friends say, "Allison, I had no idea you were having such a hard time." I put on a good face, and I isolated myself in doing so.

Growing up, I was bullied a lot. To save myself from the hurt, I became very quiet and internal. It felt easier to be by myself than to be rejected again. Yet the longer I have been walking with the Lord, the more He has begun to heal those wounds by showing me His own. He risked bearing it all on the Cross, even though some would still reject Him, because the love He had to share was worth the pain. He has been showing me lately how deep His love for me is, and as He fills me with His love, I am given the courage to be more vulnerable.

Love is worth the pain. I have learned to open up about my struggles and insecurities, and in return, others have shared theirs with me. We are heard, we are known, and we are loved, because we have made ourselves vulnerable. Vulnerability leads to authentic love. Love reduces the tendency to compare and be envious. Love builds up the body of Christ.

My hope and prayer, dear fellow mother, is that you will be encouraged by my vulnerability to open up to the mothers in your own neighborhood, church, and school. Invite them into your messy home and pray with each other for healing for the wounds that still hurt. Share a meal, start a moms' group or an exercise class, watch each other's kids for date nights. Let's rebuild the village into the one called the Kingdom of God.

9

Afterward—Looking Back

When I look into the future, I am frightened,
But why plunge into the future?
Only the present moment is precious to me,
As the future may never enter my soul at all.
It is no longer in my power,
To change, correct or add to the past;
For neither sages nor prophets could do that.
And so, what the past has embraced I must
  entrust to God.
O present moment, you belong to me, whole
  and entire.
I desire to use you as best I can.
And although I am weak and small,
You grant me the grace of your omnipotence.
And so, trusting in Your mercy,
I walk through life like a little child,
Offering You each day this heart
Burning with love for Your greater glory.[43]

[43] Saint Faustina Kowalska, *Divine Mercy*, no. 4.

Baby and Beyond

As I write this, my oldest is eight, and my youngest is two. I am
not nursing. I am sleeping through the night. I'm finally out of a
postpartum fog and feel more clear-headed than I have in years,
and I am grateful for this. But looking back gives perspective,
and that's what I wanted to offer in this book.

Looking back, there wasn't a "perfect time" to have kids.
Whether it was financial insecurities or mental health issues,
we welcomed all our children in seemingly inconvenient times.
But the truth is, I've needed these kids to overcome the struggles
I faced. I would not be who I am today without them, because
their arrivals radically changed my life in so many ways, forcing
me to confront my fears and weaknesses while opening my heart
up to greater, selfless love. And so I continually thank God that
He saw me fit to be their mother and that He gives me the grace
to accept this work of motherhood.

When Timothy was a baby, I was invited to join a "Well-Read
Mom" book club. Working part-time with a baby, I exclaimed,
"I can barely find time to shower, let alone read a book!" That
was almost eight years ago, and this year I did join a book club.
The paradox is that I have more time to read now, even though
I have more children than I did back then.

Postpartum is a season. It does not last forever, but it is profound. The way you live, sleep, and even pray changes. Just as in
autumn, when the seed falls from the tree and dies, the postpartum season shows us how much we need Christ because we don't
have it all together. We are broken, empty, exhausted. We have
to die to self. But come spring, the seed brings forth new growth,
not only literally, in terms of the baby you are raising, but also
in the spiritual life, as God is able to speak to you in new ways.

I used to get so mad at those older ladies who would tell me
to enjoy this time because it goes by fast. You mean you want

me to *enjoy* the night feedings and spit-up all over my shirt? A day can seem like forever and blend in with other days when you have a newborn. After having a few babies, though, I'm starting to get what they mean. "The days are long, but the years are short," the saying goes. I still won't miss the spit up, but it's important to savor those moments in a "you don't get this moment back" sort of way. I don't have to *enjoy* the late nights or exploding diapers, but I do have to lean into them. God meets us in the present moment. That doesn't mean that the now isn't hard, but it's all we've got.

"O life so dull and monotonous, how many treasures you contain! When I look at everything with the eyes of faith, no two hours are alike, and the dullness and monotony disappear. The grace which is given me in this hour will not be repeated in the next. It may be given me again, but it will not be the same grace."[44]

Hope

A few months ago, the kids began getting sick, one at a time. Hoarse throats, miserable coughs, fevers, waking up in the night. All the kids needed medicine, steam, blankets, lots of water, and sleep. After a week of this, I was exhausted from taking care of them and succumbed to a week of being sick myself. One day I couldn't even get out of bed. The kids watched hours upon hours of TV and after two weeks, the house was a wreck, and I had piles of laundry to catch up on. The state of exhaustion and the feeling of being overwhelmed by responsibilities reminded me of those postpartum days. It seemed as if I just couldn't catch

[44] Ibid., no. 31.

up or meet the needs of my kids. I laughed as I said to myself, "Basically, postpartum is like being sick for a year." Sure, there are good days, when you have it together, but there are lots of days when you feel as if the responsibilities are piling up and you just can't get ahead of it.

Like sickness, though, the postpartum period doesn't last. If I could go back and do postpartum all over again, I'd be gentler on myself. I'd announce survival mode, lower my expectations, not try to be "super mom," ask for help, and take naps. I'd also not fret over every decision I made, wondering if that one action has the potential to screw up my child forever (because now I know, it usually doesn't).

Now, when I look around and see my messy house, I don't (always) chide myself for being a terrible homemaker. I see the mess, and I am able to smile in gratitude that the mess is a sign of a full life. It means we were playing and exploring and learning! Cleaning it up doesn't have to be an overwhelming task; it just has to be one foot forward (and as the kids get older, they can help!).

Finally, I wish I could say that I have achieved balance between physical, mental, and spiritual health; between time for my husband, my kids, and myself, and now I've got it all together. But I don't. I wish there was a secret formula to follow in order to do it right the first time. Yet, deep inside, I know that the struggle, the failing, and the getting back up again is exactly what God is using to mold me into the person He created me to be. And so I keep struggling, I keep leaning on God's mercy, and therein lies the hope that one day I will be perfected in heaven.

About the Author

Allison Auth is a writer and blogger who lives in Denver with her husband and four children. After graduating from Franciscan University of Steubenville, she worked in youth ministry and marriage preparation until dedicating herself to the homeschooling of her children. Having gone through four postpartum experiences, she is passionate about sharing her knowledge and bringing hope to those struggling in their vocation to motherhood.

Sophia Institute

Sophia Institute is a nonprofit institution that seeks to nurture the spiritual, moral, and cultural life of souls and to spread the Gospel of Christ in conformity with the authentic teachings of the Roman Catholic Church.

Sophia Institute Press fulfills this mission by offering translations, reprints, and new publications that afford readers a rich source of the enduring wisdom of mankind.

Sophia Institute also operates the popular online resource CatholicExchange.com. *Catholic Exchange* provides world news from a Catholic perspective as well as daily devotionals and articles that will help readers to grow in holiness and live a life consistent with the teachings of the Church.

In 2013, Sophia Institute launched Sophia Institute for Teachers to renew and rebuild Catholic culture through service to Catholic education. With the goal of nurturing the spiritual, moral, and cultural life of souls, and an abiding respect for the role and work of teachers, we strive to provide materials and programs that are at once enlightening to the mind and ennobling to the heart; faithful and complete, as well as useful and practical.

Sophia Institute gratefully recognizes the Solidarity Association for preserving and encouraging the growth of our apostolate over the course of many years. Without their generous and timely support, this book would not be in your hands.

www.SophiaInstitute.com
www.CatholicExchange.com
www.SophiaInstituteforTeachers.org

Sophia Institute Press® is a registered trademark of Sophia Institute.
Sophia Institute is a tax-exempt institution as defined by the
Internal Revenue Code, Section 501(c)(3). Tax ID 22-2548708.